TURNING INTO ME

MY INTUITIVE JOURNEY THROUGH SUPERIOR CANAL DEHISCENCE SYNDROME

LAUREN FOLLONI

TURNING INTO ME: My Intuitive Journey Through Superior Canal Dehiscence Syndrome

ISBN: 979-8-9877281-0-9

Cover design by A-Schmidt.com

For Avery

CONTENTS

INTRODUCTION

This book details my experience with Superior Canal Dehiscence Syndrome (SCDS), a rare inner ear condition that causes hearing and balance problems. To conquer SCDS, I had to develop and listen to my own intuition. Through this journey, I learned that only I knew what I needed and that the answers to all my questions were already inside me.

I hope this book will help to raise awareness of this specific syndrome but also shine a light on what it's like to live with any invisible illness. There's a world out there full of people feigning to look and act "normal" as we walk through our daily lives. Some of us have SCDS. Others have migraines, depression, heart conditions, allergies, multiple sclerosis, anxiety, or another invisible illness. Chances are you encounter at least one person, more likely dozens, living with an invisible illness every day.

If you are living with an invisible illness or disability, I see you. I am with you. No matter the challenges you are facing, there is a light within you that the world needs. Keep thriving and share your story. You are not alone.

If you are living with SCDS, this book is for you. I understand your daily struggle, and I'm sorry for your pain. I hope reading my story will provide you with more comfort, less isolation, and helpful tools for navigating your SCDS journey. You are strong. You can do this.

If you love someone with an invisible illness or disability, I also see you, and I thank you for the love and kindness you bring to our world. I hope this book helps you to better understand your loved one and the unique challenges they face.

If you don't have any experience with invisible illness but do have a yearning to find yourself, and listen to yourself above all else, I hope you find hope and strength in these pages. You are wise already. Your intuition is ready and waiting for you to summon it.

1

SICK

"I am out with lanterns, looking for myself."
– Emily Dickinson

I SCARLET LETTER

A hole in the head. In hindsight, it sounds like it would be a pretty simple medical diagnosis, but, hey, what do I know? I'm no doctor. As it turns out, nothing could be more wrong. At age thirty-six, I was forced to take my health into my own hands, and in my quest to identify the noise suddenly overtaking my right ear (and my life!), I discovered the most intimate truths about myself. I learned how to listen, literally, to myself and no one else. My body. My mind. My intuition. And in this listening, I heard the truth that ultimately set me free. The answers were all there. I just had to turn in, tune in, and listen.

My health began to decline in early 2020. At that point, I had been in a relationship for eighteen months, after being single for fifteen years and raising my son by myself. My boyfriend and I were both in new jobs, and we were preparing to buy a house together for us and our two kids, my son, and his daughter. My world was changing in scary but exciting ways. My son was nearing the end of his high school years, and, as he raced toward adulthood, I was awakening to the fact that I had never experienced my adulthood without him! I knew that the next chapter of my life would have to focus on understanding my own wants and needs as a human, a woman, not just as a mother. I knew I would be starting a new chapter; I just didn't expect it to start with a medical mystery.

I woke up one morning distracted by constant noise in my right ear, as though I had water trapped in my head. It was March in New England, the beginning of Spring and allergy season. Assuming the annoying and persistent noise was an allergy symptom, I took up my daily medication regimen. I pushed the noise to the background of my life, planning for it to be gone within a couple of weeks. After all, we all had much more significant concerns in March of 2020.

As the world began grappling with the early days of the global COVID-19 pandemic, I was no exception. I was just six months into my new job. I was in a leadership position on a college campus. Now proudly working for my alma mater, I was supervising four teams and over 100 employees, checking several boxes on my professional bucket list. So, in March 2020, I had no time for noise in my ear. I was overseeing the operations of my teams as we moved our student support programs online; I was also parenting a seventeen-year-old high school junior as he took to his bedroom for weeks, and eventually months, of remote learning. He was robbed of so many of life's precious high school milestones. My heart ached for him, but as usual, I dove headfirst into my work. By putting my job first, I was putting my son first. That's how I saw it. I was providing for him.

When I was nineteen, I earned a scarlet letter[1]—and the overwhelming shame that came with it—by becoming a single teenage mother to my sweet baby boy (now a grown man). The first time I gazed into his big, chocolate-brown eyes, the opposite of my cool blue ones, I promised myself that shame would only be mine to bear. My son wouldn't feel that shame. I would mold myself into a model mother for him. He would never experience the condescending comments and sideways glances I endured throughout my young pregnancy.

Before I turned twenty-five, I had collected a bachelor's degree, a teaching license, and a graduate degree. Before thirty-five, a second graduate degree, a social work license, and a promising professional trajectory. I owned a condo and two dogs. I juggled work and single parenthood, challenging myself to be both mother and father to my young son as we grew up together, our little family of two. I squeezed a lot of work in Monday to Friday and spent my evenings and weekends in my son's world, the hockey rink, watching him do what he loves.

From the time I became a mother, every action I took revolved around ridding myself of the heavy shame I was cloaked in as a teenage parent. I was engulfed in the flames of my past; white-hot heat burned at my core, driving me to amass as many material and professional accomplishments as humanly possible. Stamping out my demons, ensuring they were not inherited by my son, was my life's work. That promise I made to him as I cradled him in my arms the very first time mattered more than anything else. I did it for him. I did it for the world. I did it to shut them all up and give my son a mom to be proud of, not embarrassed by. To give him legitimacy that no one could ever steal from him, no matter the age difference between us or the marital status of his mother. He deserved at least that, and, *wow*, I really was doing it! Even now, twenty years later, people still tell me how impressive I was, how successful I was. I soaked it in, feeling that I worked harder than any other mother ever would. That's all I needed, or so I thought.

Then, suddenly, there was this noise in my head. Suddenly, life was telling me a different story. This story forced me to ask myself who I was, what I needed, and why. Questions I had never contemplated before. Suddenly, I started wondering why my life revolved around these external forces, this shame other people had laid on my shoulders. *Why did I so readily accept this scarlet letter? Did I even like this career I was so proud of? Was my son actually proud of me? Was I proud of myself? Was I happy? Gasp!* That's not a question teenage mothers are allowed to ask. Instead, we are condemned as outsiders, suffering the consequences of our supposedly irresponsible, yet wildly common, teenage sexual relationships. Teenage mothers seek redemption, not happiness.

I have believed this bullshit for twenty years.

II STINGING DISAPPOINTMENT

The hole in my head, the lonely hell it wrought upon my life for two years, and the awakening I have experienced as a result. That's the real story here.

You have figured out by now that the noise in my ear had nothing to do with allergies, but it took an excruciatingly long time for that to be confirmed. Try as I did to will it away with allergy pills, nasal sprays, and eardrops, the noise in my right ear never went away. Two months after it started, I finally broke down and went to a doctor. Seeing most doctors' offices as a waste of time and money, I opted for the local urgent care, where I received disappointing news: my ear was completely healthy, no sign of fluid in the ear or an ear infection. Hearing you are perfectly healthy when you know something isn't right feels awful. It stings. To placate me more than anything else, the doctor agreed that I might be suffering from particularly bad seasonal allergies and suggested that I switch medications and add a third one into the mix for good measure. And with that, I was off to buy some stock in allergy medications and continue (unsuccessfully) ignoring the insatiable noise in my ear.

Life went on, our first COVID summer passed, the noise in my ear persisted, and four months later, I found myself back in an urgent care clinic. This time I chose the urgent care located within my primary care physician's (PCP) office in the hopes that I might receive elevated care or concern, this being my second doctor's appointment with the same complaint and now six months of enduring constant noise in my ear. Obviously, something was wrong. I just needed to go to my PCP's office for the answer. And so I went, and so I was disappointed again.

I very much enjoyed this doctor's visit, though. She was kind and attentive, but she was also honest. Spending maybe three minutes in the room with me, she told me (now for the second time) that my ear appeared completely healthy, no sign of fluid or infection. She gave me a referral to see an ear, nose, & throat (ENT) specialist and sent me on my way.

Health insurance being the racket that it is, turns out I couldn't see the ENT my doctor referred me to. This meant I was on my own to find a specialist to see. With a few recommendations from friends, I was able to secure an appointment at a well-respected ENT office close to my home that did accept my health insurance. This felt like my first win.

On September 11, 2020, I stepped into an ENT's office for the first time in my life. This date has meaning to every American, perhaps to the entire world. For me, it's tattooed on my heart. I was eighteen years old on September 11, 2001, living in a college dormitory in lower Manhattan when terrorists brutalized America, taking nearly 3,000 innocent lives and forever changing mine. I lived and attended school three blocks from the World Trade Center, so close that you could not see the tops of the twin towers from my twelfth-story bedroom window.

I thought September 11 was going to be the last day of my life. Instead, it became the first. A fork in the road that chose me and gave me no other option but to face the fear and the trauma it left in its wake and forge a personal peace and healing from it. Each year on that date, I spend the day in solemnity. I listen to the ceremonies in New York, taking in the names of every man, woman, and child we lost that day. I mourn for them even though I never met them. I remember my own experiences—naivety, terror, horror—from that day and the weeks following the tragedy and do what I can to ensure that we never forget. But in 2020, I didn't do that. Instead, I visited an ENT's office. This, my willingness to schedule a doctor's appointment on this date, was one of my first signals that my ear was becoming a bigger disruption than I was outwardly acknowledging.

I enjoyed this doctor's visit as well. The ENT was clearly experienced. His office had the diplomas and framed newspaper articles to prove it. He was kind, attentive, and thorough, setting me up for two separate appointments on the same day, which actually became three. I began the appointments by meeting with an audiologist for a hearing test. I then met with the ENT, where I tried to explain the noise "like water and pressure," I said, in my ear. He asked me a series of questions. He stuck an endoscope so far up my nose it went down my throat! He sent me for impromptu allergy testing, asking a colleague to squeeze me into their day since I was already there. I was thrilled with this service! I was having tests done. I was having a conversation with a specialist. I was invited to stick around and see him again after the allergy testing to determine my treatment plan together. This was exactly the type of care and attention I had been hoping for coming into this appointment.

Hours later, I was met with my third dose of stinging disappointment. The ENT told me my ear was perfectly healthy and diagnosed me with severe allergies and gastroesophageal reflux disease (GERD). He added two prescriptions to my existing medications and sent me on my way with instructions to come back in one month for a followup. I accepted this next appointment as a challenge. I gave myself one month to figure out what I was doing wrong here. I had now seen five healthcare providers: two urgent care physicians, an audiologist, an allergist, and an ENT!

And everyone said my ear was fine. *Was it fine? What is going on here? Am I losing my mind?*

I came to realize I had two choices: 1. Accept that I was dealing with something no one else could see or hear and find a way to communicate it to my doctors, or 2. Accept the fact that I must be insane and imagining this noise in my ear. Maybe I had finally cracked up after all the years of pressure I was putting on myself to be the perfect mother. I was finally succumbing to the scarlet letter. It was stealing my mind.

But no! Damn it, no! The noise really was there. I was convinced. I had to convince others now. I had to show up for myself. I had to turn in, tune in, and listen to myself.

Over the next month, my distraction with my right ear flourished into an obsession. Instead of pushing the noise to the back of my mind, I placed it at the center of my life. I tuned in and invited it in to live my daily life with me so I could understand it better and deliver its message to my doctor. This noise was with me constantly. Sometimes it was a deafening roar. Other times just a whisper. It hadn't responded to any treatment attempts to date, so I knew it had nothing to do with my allergies. It was louder when I was very stressed. It was most loud when I was active or exercising or when I drank alcohol. It wasn't tinnitus. It wasn't a ringing sound at all. It was persistent every night while I lay in bed trying to sleep. *Boom boom boom.* An endless loop of *boom boom boom.*

And then, out of nowhere, a revelation. It was my heartbeat. Yes! Absolutely yes. It was my heartbeat. When my son was born, there was a popular teddy bear at the time. The teddy bear made a heartbeat sound. The theory being that it was comforting to infants as they slept in their bassinets, adjusting to the world outside of the mother's womb. That teddy bear is exactly what the noise in my ear sounded like. *Boom boom boom.* Directly in sync with my pulse. I had cracked the puzzle—and to confirm it, I raced up and down a flight of stairs several times to make it as loud as I possibly could. *BOOM BOOM BOOM!* My head screamed in response to the physical exertion. *Yes, yes! This is my heartbeat.* It's loud and clear, and it's loudest when my heart is pumping hard. Now I can tell the doctors exactly what I'm hearing. Now the doctors will know what to do.

It took me that whole month to figure out the noise was my heartbeat, so my follow-up appointment came quickly. I bounced into the doctor's office, full of optimism. Today was the day, seven months later, that they would tell me what was wrong, and we would get to work fixing it. This time I didn't see the doctor, though. He had assigned my appointment to a Physician's Assistant (PA). I like to think of myself as young despite really being middle-aged if I'm honest, but this guy? This guy really was young. But he was also very kind and attentive, just like the doctor had been, and I'm a social worker, for crying out loud. I like to stay open-minded, and I know this man had completed a lot of specialized training. So, I took a deep breath, promised myself to see this through, and shared my revelation with him. "It's my heartbeat that I'm hearing!"

His response was a couple of rapid-fire questions trying to confirm that it really was my heartbeat I was hearing. Satisfied with my responses, he gave my noise a name. *Pulsatile tinnitus.* To me, it's a weird name since it's not much like the tinnitus we commonly think of at all. Pulsatile tinnitus, a form of objective tinnitus, is when the patient can hear their own blood flow, through veins near the ear. The more common tinnitus we hear about, like ringing in the ears, does not have an anatomical origin, it is phantom noise often linked to hearing loss. This is called subjective tinnitus. According to the American Tinnitus Association[2], tinnitus is quite common, affecting up to 15% of the American population, but less than 1% of those cases are objective tinnitus, like what many SCDS patients are experiencing when they hear their heartbeat.

The PA quickly explained that a brain MRI is necessary when a patient reports pulsatile tinnitus, then said he wanted to bring the doctor in for a moment, and he left the room briskly. I sat there alone with this news. It dawned on me that maybe I didn't really want to know what might be causing this noise. For the first time, I was afraid of the underlying problem.

When they returned, the doctor explained to me that pulsatile tinnitus can be a sign of brain tumor or aneurysm. For that reason, they would be ordering an MRI of my brain to "rule them out." They provided me with instructions for scheduling that appointment, explained that it would take time because our crooked (my honest opinion) healthcare system needs to approve the MRI before I was allowed to schedule it, and said I would receive a phone call from them with the results in the days following the MRI. All this would take several weeks at minimum. In this ten-minute appointment, I went from flying high with optimism because I had finally figured out how to communicate what I was hearing to a numbing fear that I would learn in the coming weeks that I had a life-threatening brain condition. A mother battling a brain tumor cannot provide for her son. A mother dead from a brain aneurysm would be the worst-case scenario for my boy. It was impossible not to go there in my head. Neither of these could be my reality. Something else was happening.

III "GOOD NEWS"

The next five months dragged on at a snail's pace. The first MRI passed. Normal results. "Good news!" the PA said to me on the phone after three weeks of waiting that might as well have been an eternity. "There is no sign of tumor, aneurysm, or stroke in your brain. Let's schedule a follow-up again in three months." Yes, yes, rationally, I understand this is good news, but again I was left with stinging disappointment. Back to square one. No answers. More waiting.

I still had this constant *boom boom boom* in my ear, and as I remained tuned in to the noise in my head—desperately seeking more information I could clearly communicate to doctors – I came to acknowledge more and more symptoms. Some of them were new, but some had been part of my life for many years, and many of them were very odd. I'm a lifelong headache sufferer, but specifically, I suffered from cluster headaches around my right eye. I began to wonder if there was some connection between these right-side headaches and the noise being in my right ear. I had also developed motion sickness in the last few years.

Exploring my symptoms became a second job. As I took daily inventory of myself, checking in with my body, I began noticing many changes. I could not tolerate surround sound from the TV because it caused pain in my ears. Similarly, I was finding it hard to track motion across the television screen, which I noticed while watching Harry Potter movies with the constant motion of some object or another flying through the air. Tracking motion like this produced an uncomfortable sensation in my eyes that made me just want to keep them closed.

I was also having extreme difficulty at work. Historically, learning a new job was never an arduous challenge for me, regardless of how substantial my workload or how great the learning curve was. This time, though, was proving to be much different at my new job. Now in this role for a full year, I still encountered situations daily that felt difficult. I was struggling to learn and keep up cognitively, like my brain was operating at half-capacity. I soon found I needed a nap in the middle of most workdays just to get through the day.

Simultaneously, my threshold for noise was steadily decreasing. Ordinary noises caused me great discomfort—the dog barking, the sound of silverware tinkling when emptying the dishwasher, the clinking of stacking plates, television. Noise became sharp and painful, and it was everywhere.

Like my revelation about pulsatile tinnitus, through deep and silent introspection, I realized that I was also hearing my eyeballs move. *Crunch crunch crunch* as my eyes surveyed the world around me, every eye movement resulting in a sound like crunching snow beneath your feet. Walking through a mall with my son, I noticed that the environmental noise of people talking in the wide-open spaces was deafening. I was so overwhelmed by the noise inside, I couldn't hear my son, walking directly beside me, speaking to me. I was hearing everything and nothing all at the same time.

I would tell my loved ones these odd symptoms, and their faces would strain with sympathy and bewilderment. I knew they wanted to believe me, but I also knew that I *looked* perfectly healthy, and I must have sounded insane. Friends and family would try to reassure me with reminders that everyone was struggling and suffering. Between COVID-19 concerns, social isolation, remote work and school, civil and political unrest, and racial injustice in our streets, life was hard for us all, and I knew that was true. Stress levels were at record highs, including my own. But I also knew I was experiencing something else. Something on top of all that. And I was in it alone. No one else could understand.

I began to cry every day. Depression and anxiety set in as I fought what felt like a desperate losing battle to understand why I was losing control of my body, of my life. The experience of falling apart on the inside while I looked the same on the outside ravaged my mind and stole my peace. I was lost. At this low moment, I made a second promise to myself. This time it had nothing to do with motherhood. This time I promised to believe in myself and never to give up on myself. I knew my body was sick. I would honor it, defend it, and do whatever I could to heal it.

Eventually, those three months between check-ins passed, and I found myself back in the ENT's office, meeting with the PA again. It was now clear that my case had been permanently assigned to the PA. I presumed my "normal" MRI results meant that the doctor felt comfortable handing my straightforward case of allergies and GERD over to a PA. I knew I wasn't a basic case, though. I knew that I had something much bigger going on. I just didn't know what it was or how to get their attention. I began coaching myself before doctor appointments, giving myself a pep talk to steel my nerves and mentally prepare to advo-cate for myself in the face of a medical system designed to minimize valid patient concerns. I would send messages back and forth with my best friends to puff myself up and borrow courage from them. They came with me in spirit, keeping me strong and holding me accountable, knowing I wanted to relay a story back to them that I was proud of when I left the doctor's office. I would not allow myself to be minimized or silenced.

At this next appointment, I just regurgitated my newfound facts. All the gory details I had been collecting day in and day out, including that I was certain I was hearing my eyeballs move. The PA's response was, "Wow, that's crazy! I've never heard of that." I began advocating for myself as best I could. I asked him what our next steps could be. He explained that he could request a second MRI; this one is called an MRA, noted by the presence of IV-injected dye, which shows your blood vessels in more detail. This MRA would again be looking for tumors, or any type of vascular issue in my brain, that the dye contrast could pick up if it was missed in the first MRI. Undergoing another long and loud MRI was dead last on my wish list, but I didn't know what else to do. I would take any test they would give. So, I hopped on the health insurance merry-go-round again, waited several weeks, and then scheduled the first available MRA appointment. By the time I underwent the MRA testing, I had been sick for eleven months, and I was more lost than ever before.

I stumbled my way through this next disappointment when the PA called to tell me the "good news" that my results came back normal again. Everything is normal and healthy, he told me. But it wasn't! I wasn't okay! I was crying every day. I was becoming a shell of a person. I could muster up enough energy each day to drag myself through a day of work (at home, in my pajamas), cook dinner for my family, then go straight to bed. My relationships with my boyfriend and his daughter, as well as my son, grew distant despite sharing the same house. Being a typical teenager, my son was focused on his own challenges. Since he was finishing high school during a pandemic, there were many—and I think I was pretty successful in shielding him from my crazy symptoms. There was no denying, though, that I was sick, and I was acting very differently now.

We added a little stuffed octopus toy that could be turned inside out to our household. One side was yellow and smiley; the other side was red and mad. This was my silent signal to my family of what kind of day I was having. I lost all capacity to speak my needs or express my feelings without crying. It didn't take long for a signal to become unnecessary, though. Every day was a bad day. I was plummeting into the depths of hell. I understand how dramatic this sounds, but I promise you this is no exaggeration.

The PA could hear the upset in my voice as he relayed the "good" MRA results. He was incredibly kind, but we were obviously at a standstill. I was defeated. He advised me to give it time and hope that my symptoms subsided on their own. His instructions were to call in six months to schedule a follow-up appointment to see how I was doing. I hung up the phone and cried and honestly wondered how I could survive that long.

It was now winter of 2021. In four short months, my only child would be graduating from high school. I wanted to be present for this once-in-a-lifetime season of life with him, so I decided to tune out. I would stop listening to the noises in my head and do whatever I could to push it all aside and pretend I was fine like the doctors kept saying I was. At this point in my life, I had developed a strong will to persevere in the face of adversity. I owned my survivor identity like a badge of honor and lived by a mantra of resiliency. Life had already thrown me many challenges in the way of external forces to contend with—this was just the next challenge, and I would overcome this one as well because nothing was more important than being the best mother I could be. I willed myself to harness the power of my mind and transcend the noise.

That lasted about two weeks.

In late February of 2021, one year into the global pandemic, I was invited to speak to the university's Board of Trustees and recognize the great work my department had accomplished that year. This was an honor I was thrilled to accept on behalf of the exceptional staff I worked with each day. I was keenly aware of how my colleagues had risen to the tremendous challenge of moving our work online, finding new and innovative ways to support college students through this sudden and substantial shift in education, and managing their own daily challenges as humans living through a pandemic. Moreover, I couldn't help but feel as though I had let my employees down over this last year, as I struggled with the noise in my head and knew I was not giving my usual 110% at work like I normally would—and because I got sick so soon after becoming a new leader in the department, they really didn't know that old version of me at all. I was desperate to let them hear how proud I was of them. I wrote a speech that I hoped would accurately convey to my teams, and to the university's highest leadership ranks, just how impressive their work had been and how deserving they were of this formal recognition.

The meeting was held remotely via video conference. When it was my turn to speak, I sat up straight, unmuted my microphone, and confidently launched into my speech, projecting my voice loud and strong. Immediately, I was hit by an equally loud sound *inside* my head. Every word I spoke was being amplified in my right ear, bouncing around inside my skull with a loud, distorted noise like microphone feedback. It hit me physically, like a ton of bricks, knocking me backward in my chair, leaving me reeling for a moment. Like a reflex, to make the noise stop, I paused for a beat of silence. My mind was reeling. *What was that?!*

I couldn't let that question matter in that moment, though. I sat up again and forced my way through the speech. With every word, my own distorted voice rang back through my right ear like a demonic echo. I was hearing myself twice. And I could *feel* my voice. Vibrations jumped up and down the right side of my skull with every word that came out of my mouth. I was crumbling to pieces inside with the realization that I wasn't going to be able to defeat this thing with my thoughts alone. I needed a diagnosis. I needed medical care. Something was wrong. On the outside, I did my best to smile through the speech and deliver this moment of acknowledgment to my staff.

A week later, I was sitting back in the ENT's office, across from the PA, telling him I had figured out what was wrong. I had diagnosed myself.

IV LISTENING TO MYSELF

Autophony. The "abnormal hearing of one's own voice, breathing, and other internal sounds."[3] Autophony is what I experienced during that speech for the Board of

Trustees. My own distorted voice in my ear, amplified, unpleasant, and painful. Autophony was also my ability to hear my own eyeballs move. I could hear my eyes blink, as well. My neck creaking. My stomach digesting a meal. My footsteps. My bodily noises were ringing out inside my head, all day every day. I was coming to this realization less than two weeks after my doctor told me I was fine, and I had, in utter defeat, agreed to wait six months to see if the symptoms magically went away on their own. I was completely alone in this. If I wanted answers, I needed to find them myself.

I took to Google.

But first, I sat with myself. In silence. I asked myself if the noises were real. I asked myself if I was mentally well or if I needed psychological care. I asked myself if I was physically well. I embraced myself literally and figuratively, wrapping my body up in its own arms and telling it that I would not abandon it. I cried as I had every day in recent memory, but this time I cried peaceful tears. They were a promise of healing. I promised my body that I would not ask it to be broken like this, and I wouldn't force it to be sick. I promised my mind that I would trust it. Then I went to work, ready to do whatever it took to find my diagnosis.

I'm a social worker, which means that I am a trained diagnostician. I understand how incredibly difficult it is to receive a patient's oral report of various symptoms I have never experienced myself and, with this limited information, track down an accurate diagnosis. Diagnosing an ailment is complicated, difficult, and requires trial and error. I knew that much going in. Obviously, I didn't attend medical school, and I didn't possess the medical knowledge of any doctor, certainly not of an ENT specialist, but I wasn't going to let that stop me.

I had now been sick for a full year and had written a list of twenty-six symptoms I was experiencing on a regular basis, most of them daily. So, I pulled out that list and went through each symptom one by one. For each symptom, I asked myself two questions: 1. Did I explain this to the doctor? 2. How did the doctor respond? After reviewing all twenty-six, one of them leaped off the page.

Hearing my eyeballs move was a particularly distressing symptom for me. I am an avid reader of fiction, and the reason why I love to read fiction is because it is my release from the stressors of life. It is my escapism. I lost that escape, though, when my reading became marred by the crunching noise of my eyeballs moving, scrolling across the page. Line after line of scraping, crunching noise. This was no escape for me anymore. These noises were stealing my entire life. Yet, you'll recall that when I told the doctor I was hearing my eyes move, he replied that that was "crazy" and he hadn't heard of it before. He did record it in his notes, but he swiftly changed the subject and never brought it up again. I felt very defeated at that moment and was fine to leave that feeling of defeat in the past when that appointment was over.

Now in hindsight, I realized that this was critical insight. Every other symptom I had shared with the doctor was discussed and explored. They were all dead ends, but they were all heard. This was the only exception.

So, I opened a web browser, typed "I can hear my eyes move" into the search bar, and hit Enter. A BBC News article entitled "Man Cured of Hearing His Eyeballs

Move"[4] immediately popped up. I clicked on the link and read a story published in 2011 about a man in England. I instantly knew. In a few short minutes, I was sure I knew what was wrong with me. Without the magic of the internet, I would probably still be suffering today, searching for a diagnosis.

V THE ANSWERS ARE WITHIN

I stuttered out loud to myself in my home office, struggling with new vocabulary words. Superior Canal Dehiscence Syndrome (SCDS). This man from England had all my symptoms. He described a dull headache on one side, his voice reverberating through his head, some dizziness, blurry vision, hearing his own heartbeat, and hearing his eyes move. And best of all, this man had been cured!

I had been seeing doctors for ten months in search of an elusive diagnosis. I had brought myself to hell and back, growing more and more afraid that I might actually be physically fine but going insane. But here it was. A valid medical diagnosis: SCDS. I had just diagnosed myself in under five minutes! I grabbed my phone and scheduled the first available ENT appointment.

I floated into that ENT's office the following week. I printed the article (and a few more webpages I had found) and delivered them to the PA, saying with as much confidence as I could muster, "I think this is what I have. Have you heard of this?" He knew what SCDS was but told me it is a very rare condition and that it was unlikely I had it.

The feeling I had at that moment can't be described. Absolute dejection. It took every cell in my body to gather the courage to push forward with the conversation and make sure it wasn't dismissed.

Deep breaths. Turning in. Collecting myself. Promising my body I would take care of it. Telling myself to be strong in this moment. I can do this!

I told the PA I understood that this was a very rare condition, but I at least needed to have the appropriate testing to rule it out. I told him that my research said a CT scan was necessary to test for SCDS. I asked him if I could at least have a CT scan to rule it out. He agreed. And once again, I hopped on the health insurance merry-go-round, waiting several weeks for the CT scan to be approved and scheduled. Again, I was told to expect a phone call on the days after the test with my results.

After my MRI tests, I learned that no one was in any rush to contact you if your scan yields normal results. I waited up to a week for the results of both MRIs, so I tried to steel my nerves and find some patience going into the CT scan. I was boiling over with anxiety. I felt it in my soul that I had SCDS. I knew I was right. But the PA's voice nagged at me constantly, telling me how rare SCDS was and that it was unlikely I had it. If I was wrong, if I didn't have SCDS, if I had to go back to the drawing board, well, it was just unthinkable. Instead, I chose to trust in myself. Listen to my intuition. I was certain I was correct on this.

My CT scan was completed around 6:30 pm on Tuesday, March 16, 2021. I hoped to get a phone call sometime that week with the results so I wouldn't have to wait through the weekend. It came the very next morning before lunchtime! Just three business hours had passed since my CT scan was completed. My phone lit up with the ENT's phone number, and I heard that kind, attentive PA's voice on the line. "I'm sorry," he said, "You were right." He told me what I already knew: the CT scan did suggest a dehiscence (hole) at the top of my superior semicircular canal, and the only available treatment, he said, is a "fairly invasive" surgery. Next, he would provide me with a referral to another specialist, this time in Boston, as his office was unequipped for cases like mine.

My soul sang.

Second to meeting my son, this moment was my proudest accomplishment. Through this, I learned my most important lesson. I can turn inward for the answers I seek and let my intuition guide the way. As I inched closer to a diagnosis over all those months, I wanted to give up many times. I even had doctors recommending that I give up looking for a diagnosis. My intuition propelled me forward, though, and gave me the wisdom and strength I needed to partner with doctors and advocate for my needs until we finally uncovered the answers together.

2

SCDS

"The way out is in."

– Thich Nhat Hanh

I UNDERSTANDING SUPERIOR CANAL DEHISCENCE SYNDROME (SCDS)

To understand SCDS, and what it's like to live with it, you first need some basic knowledge. Let's begin with the name. What is the name? How do you say it? What does it mean? All-important questions to start with.

You've noticed that I call it Superior Canal Dehiscence Syndrome. Dehiscence sounds like da-HISS-ins, and basically, it means hole. So, someone with a dehiscence of their superior canal has a hole in the bone surrounding their superior canal. By tacking the word syndrome onto the end, we are saying this person is experiencing symptoms because of that hole. SCDS is the name I've always used to describe my condition. However, there are slight variations used across the medical field, such as: Superior Semicircular Canal Dehiscence (SSCD), Superior Canal Dehiscence (SCD), or even Semicircular Canal Dehiscence. As you can see, these are all variations of similar names. The majority of SCDS patients have a dehiscence of the superior canal, which I assume explains why it's in the name. However, some people have a dehiscence affecting another ear canal (horizontal or posterior), so you can understand why removing "superior" from the name of the syndrome would feel more applicable for those patients. No matter what name your doctor uses, you should be aware of them all if you're conducting internet research.

When it comes to helping loved ones understand the condition, the name can be a surprisingly big hurdle. It's a lot of words, a lot of syllables, and it lacks clarity for your average layperson. It *requires* explanation. Just using an acronym doesn't relieve that challenge, of course, because an acronym doesn't offer any information about the condition it describes, but, frankly, it's just easier to say. My advice is to pick the acronym that best works for you, find a quick way to explain what it means to your loved ones, and stick with using just that one name. Then, use the name often in conversation with family and friends so that everyone can get comfortable with the key terms. I felt hurt and invalidated when my loved ones could not even remember the name of the condition that was stealing my life. SCDS was consuming my life for a long time, but the people closest to me couldn't even name it. It's not their fault, but that didn't prevent the hurt. In hindsight, I realize I could've made sure I took the time to teach them the name so that we could all have had a shared language.

An understanding of SCDS also requires knowledge of how the inner ear works. This is no easy feat as this tiny, delicate system (only the size of a quarter!) is vastly complex. The inner ear houses two critical functions: hearing and balance. You might recall from fifth-grade science class that we have three semicircular canals in our inner ear. People with SCDS have a dehiscence, or a hole, in one of those semicircular canals.

Hearing is created when sound travels into our outer ear, through the middle ear, and ends up in the inner ear, where these semicircular canals are located. Finally, it enters the cochlea, which is filled with fluid that vibrates in response to sound, sending an electrical impulse to our brain, which creates hearing. So, in a person with SCDS, this abnormal hole in the inner ear allows the patient to hear noises they shouldn't be able to, namely from within their own body.

Our body's ability to maintain balance is controlled by the vestibular system, which also happens to be housed inside the inner ear. The vestibular system uses signals it receives from the semicircular canals to understand when and how our head is moving. This sensory input allows our eyes and brain to work together with the vestibular system to understand where our body is in space and enables us to remain upright and maintain balance. When our vestibular functioning is not working properly, we can experience vertigo, a sensation as though we are, or the world is, spinning or moving. We can also experience dizziness, which is like vertigo but not the same. Dizziness is a more general term used to describe feelings of imbalance, lightheadedness, motion sickness, etc.

SCDS is a newly identified condition. It was discovered in 1995, when I was in junior high, by Dr. Lloyd Minor, a surgeon at Johns Hopkins. At this point, I want to ask you to pause with me for a moment of reflection. Please just put your book down for a moment, close your eyes, and think of the millions of people suffering from SCDS prior to 1995 and those still searching for a diagnosis even today.

A life with SCDS is a life of pain and suffering. It is an existence so barren, lonely, and isolating that it almost certainly snatches all joy from the patient's life, at least momentarily. It robs mothers of precious moments with their children, whose cries are too shrill to be too close for too long. It robs relationships of intimacy, friendships of connection, and individuals of their self-worth.

SCDS is often invisible to the naked eye and produces symptoms so shocking and peculiar to report that it's very common for patients to be referred from medical care to psychiatric care! It's not unheard of for someone with SCDS to be diagnosed with severe mental illness, including schizophrenia, when auditory symptoms are mistaken for hallucinations.

I'll likely never meet Dr. Minor, but he will always be a personal hero of mine. I have spent many hours in meditation speaking to those SCDS sufferers who came before me, who came before Dr. Minor, and whose lives were permanently stained by SCDS without ever knowing the cause of their suffering. I pray for their eternal peace, knowing that they likely did not have it in life. And while I am dismayed that SCDS is not yet better understood by doctors, I am grateful beyond measure to those specialists we do currently have. These doctors are saving lives. Mine is one of them.

Today, the predominant theory in the medical community is that many people with SCDS were either born with a hole there or these bones never fully developed in utero and were too thin from birth. So, as we age and bones naturally thin, a tiny hole sometimes forms in the area of the semicircular canals. Most often it's the superior canal. However, the dehiscence can also result from head trauma (think sports injuries, car accidents, etc.) or even an infection.

The abnormal hole can *sometimes* wreak havoc. Much to my surprise, I have learned through my research that it is possible to have a dehiscence that is inactive, meaning no symptoms are experienced even though there *is* a hole in the bone. Conversely, it's also possible to have no dehiscence—just thin bone—and experience SCDS symptoms. One of the many online lectures I watched compared this phenomenon to thin walls in an apartment building; there doesn't need to be a hole in the wall for you to hear noise from your neighbors. The same can be true for a patient with only very thin bone. (Are you starting to see why SCDS is so misunderstood and hard to diagnose? My frustration in seeking a diagnosis was more about how sick I was feeling than it was about thinking doctors didn't care or didn't want to help me. That was never my experience with any doctor I met along the way.)

In my case, though, I did have a dehiscence and it was active, resulting in a host of miserable symptoms I've already started to describe. An active dehiscence creates something doctors call a "third window phenomenon." A healthy ear has two holes where sound enters and exits.

Noise enters our middle ear through the stapes bone at the oval window and exits at the other end through something called the round window.

In a normal situation, our ear operates as a closed system, keeping the noise contained inside these tiny bony structures. But when a dehiscence is present, suddenly, there is a third window (aka hole, aka dehiscence) present. Sound can now travel in and out of this third window. This means that the hole in the semicircular canal allows noise to travel between your inner ear and your brain instead of being contained in the ear. This allows the patient to hear their own bodily noises, such as eyeball movement, heartbeat, footsteps, etc.

Sound also creates vibration as it's traveling around in the ear, and this can stimulate the fluid in the ear canals, causing problems for our vestibular system, our balance. Pressure changes can induce these balance problems as well. Everyday activities like coughing, sneezing, or even laughing can lead to dizziness or vertigo when the pressure in this delicate system is impacted. Unexpected loud noises, like fire alarms, sirens, or loud music, can do the same.

Long story short, doctors say there are two categories of symptoms associated with SCDS: 1. Auditory (Hearing), and 2. Vestibular (Balance). An SCDS patient can experience auditory symptoms, vestibular symptoms, or both. This is a critical piece of information as much misinformation and incorrect guidance seems to exist in the medical community. Many SCDS patients are told by their ENT that they cannot have SCDS because they initially report symptoms from just one category: auditory or vestibular. That is wrong! Doctors who specialize in treating SCDS patients are very clear on this. A patient can experience only auditory or only vestibular symptoms. If you encounter a doctor saying someone must have both auditory and vestibular symptoms to be diagnosed with SCDS, seek a second opinion from an SCDS specialist. As a person who is unwell, you deserve the best treatment from the most experienced provider possible.

There is much more to life with SCDS, though, even beyond the auditory and vestibular symptoms. I argue strongly that there's a third category of SCDS symptoms that I call Cognitive & Other Symptoms. Since I'm more educated on this topic than a lot of doctors—both through my lived experience and through extensive research, as well as conversations with other SCDS patients via a life-changing Facebook community I joined—I'm taking my own word for it and will talk in detail in the coming pages about these other symptoms. Their importance, specifically how common they are and how debilitating they can be, cannot be overstated. I hope that someday we will see this "other" group of symptoms more widely acknowledged and explored by the medical community.

I first noticed auditory symptoms, so I'll describe those first.

II AUDITORY SYMPTOMS

For the first year, I only experienced auditory symptoms. My first symptoms were pulsatile tinnitus (hearing my own heartbeat) and autophony (hearing my own bodily noises from within), which started as hearing my eyeballs move.

I was living with a bass drum in my ear. *BOOM BOOM BOOM!* My heartbeat was sometimes so loud that I could not hear anything else. *BOOM BOOM BOOM!* While I was trying to concentrate at work, trying to sleep at night, trying to exercise, trying to read. At times, I was so keenly aware of my heartbeat that I could actually hear the pumping in *and* out of my heart. Bah-boom bah-boom bah-boom. The wet sound of turbulent blood flow sloshed in my ear. On top of that, I could *feel* my pulse through my head, neck, and chest on the right side. Many SCDS patients report this physical sensation in addition to the sound, but doctors don't know what causes it. With every heartbeat, my right side felt a thump, and my right ear received the muffled *boom boom boom* of the pulsatile tinnitus. It was my constant companion. My primary SCDS complaint.

As you know, I eventually noticed a second noise that I could tell was *not* my heartbeat. This noise was kind of crunchy and scratchy. For a long time, I described it as ants walking around in my ear, and this was before I knew what was wrong, so the mental torment I was putting myself through imagining what could be happening inside my head was horrendous. This is when I started always carrying my phone to play music at all times. I had to try to drown out the noise. Eventually, I figured out this second noise only happened when I moved my eyes, and sounded like the crunching of snow under your feet as you walk on it.

Another auditory symptom I experienced is called hyperacusis, which is sensitivity to sound. Hyperacusis elicits sharp pain even from the most benign noises, like emptying the dishwasher or a baby crying. Not injury pain, more like the pain you experience when you hear a dog whistle or microphone feedback. Once, while at my sister's house for a family holiday gathering, my mother began emptying the silverware from the dishwasher. Pain pricked my body head to toe as I stepped behind my boyfriend and said, "She's trying to kill me with that silverware!" Bad humor aside, I found that making light of my pain was one of the only ways to invite people into my experience in a way that wouldn't further alienate me or make me sound *too* insane.

I also experienced this bizarre phenomenon where I heard everything and nothing at the same time. This mostly only happened in public (restaurants, malls, the office, full houses on holidays) where the environmental noises create a din so loud I couldn't hear the person right next to me speaking. The worst part, for me, of hyperacusis is that it produces an exaggerated startle response. When I heard an unexpected noise, my body would go into a full fight or flight response, and I would experience that burst of adrenaline that explodes from your chest and down your extremities. While lying in bed reading one night, my partner spoke unexpectedly to me, and his voice made me leap out of my skin, like a jump scare in a haunted house. I was cozy in my own bed, though, enjoying my book, totally relaxed. But my body couldn't respond normally to noise anymore. I ended up asking him to touch me before he spoke so that I could have some warning that noise would be coming.

I also experienced autophony in several other forms aside from hearing my heartbeat and my eyes move. I could hear my own distorted voice inside my head, like speaking through a kazoo. I could also *feel* my voice; there was a vibration that reverberated up and down my skull when talking. Giving presentations at work, something I often do as a manager, was about as enjoyable as sticking an ice pick in my ear. I could hear my footsteps the same way, both from the outside and inside my head. Same goes for my chewing. I was munching on a salad once, about two feet away from my partner but not looking directly at him. When I stopped chewing, he said, "No? You got nothing?" He was speaking to me while I was chewing, and I had no idea he had said anything. I could hear my neck creaking, my eyes blinking, and a bubbling sort of noise that I realized much later (from reading about others' experiences with SCDS) was the sound of my food digesting after a meal.

I also had an almost constant sensation of fullness in my head and ears. Sometimes, the fullness was isolated to my right ear, as though the ear was full of fluid and muffled. Often, though, the fullness affected my whole head, like that full, congested feeling you have during a severe head cold.

The cumulative effect of these auditory symptoms is a burning need for control. The only way to survive the onslaught of constant noise is to find ways to control your environment and protect yourself. I listened to music at every waking moment as a distraction. I changed out the kitchen cabinet hardware so it wouldn't make noise when the cabinets closed, and I replaced the heavy ceramic dinner plates with lightweight plasticware that made far less noise when stacking plates. I bought ear plugs to wear in public to take the sharp edge off the environmental noise, particularly in restaurants, but even those only helped slightly. While they dulled the pain associated with hyperacusis, they plugged my ear, which amplified my internal noises. In situations like this, I had to opt for the louder internal noises because, while loud, they didn't produce pain the way hyperacusis did.

My auditory symptoms forced a reclusive lifestyle. Leaving the house for, well, basically any reason became almost unthinkable. The cacophony of life—chit-chat at parties, surround sound in movie theaters, police or fire sirens, ordinary road traffic, concerts, public transportation, your favorite song, and even the voice of someone you love— brings pain and discomfort upon you. The only answer is to be alone. By the end of my first year living with SCDS, 90% of my life was contained to two rooms: my home office and my bedroom. My life was a shadow of what it once was, and absolutely no one could understand what I was experiencing.

III VESTIBULAR SYMPTOMS

My first year with SCDS was vestibular symptom-free. After that first year with my noisy friends, they brought their dizzy friends to the party. Most days, I would feel dizzy and lightheaded for the first hour or two of my day because mornings didn't suck enough.

It's common for SCDS sufferers to say they feel like they're on a boat. It can also be difficult to walk on surfaces that aren't smooth. A walk in the woods feels like trying to traverse one of those rickety wooden bridges in movies that span a terrifying ravine. A walking stick is often necessary, but I'd be lying if I told you I even tried to walk in the woods while sick. It's one of the many things I stopped doing when SCDS took over. In bed at night, I would often have the "spins," even when stone-cold sober. Speaking of sober, I stopped drinking alcohol altogether. When I did drink more than one drink, I would have violent vertigo. I'm talking zero-gravity, somersaults in space, complete disorientation vertigo, and deafening pulsatile tinnitus. No drink is worth that nightmare.

I also experienced discomfort while driving, including an intense desire to close my eyes because it felt hard to track the motion around me, which lots of SCDS patients describe. Moving my head back and forth quickly while driving made me feel dizzy and lightheaded. Another symptom was a feeling of being pulled backward. This was especially true for me in the shower.

In hindsight, after my SCDS diagnosis, I was even able to acknowledge some symptoms I had for several years prior. In my late twenties, I developed motion sickness. This was something I had never experienced before. Throughout childhood, I easily traveled in cars, on planes, and happily rode roller coasters, but I started experiencing consistent car sickness as an adult. Maybe this could have been an early sign of my bone thinning, a developing dehiscence.

While living with SCDS, I tuned in closely to barometric pressure each day as it most certainly had an impact on my vestibular symptoms and quality of life. Barometric pressure is the amount of pressure in the Earth's atmosphere at any given time. Tiny changes in barometric pressure cause changes in weather and, in fact, can be felt throughout the human body. You may know someone with arthritis who can predict bad weather by an increase in joint pain. When barometric pressure is low, weather is stormy, and living with SCDS is more difficult. Aural fullness was at its peak for me during periods of low barometric pressure, as well as headache, dizziness, and vertigo. Most SCDS patients I have encountered use an app to track the barometric pressure to be prepared for harder days, harder seasons. Winter is not easy, especially a particularly stormy and snowy winter.

I was fortunate. My vestibular symptoms were very minor as far as SCDS goes. I did experience them every day, but they were typically not severe or debilitating. Many SCDS sufferers must manage severe vertigo every day of their lives. So, I count my blessings in that I know my SCDS journey could have been even harder were I to have experienced extreme vestibular problems.

IV COGNITIVE & OTHER SYMPTOMS

These are the ones that, for the most part, aren't formally recognized as symptoms of SCDS, despite how debilitating, frustrating, and common they are. I know I am not alone in this. I don't know why they aren't widely acknowledged by the medical community. I can only assume it's because SCDS is simply still too unfamiliar. Much more research and education are needed.

SCDS ravages your mind. Your brain is processing overwhelming sound and sensory input every minute of every day. Your body is trying to recalibrate almost constantly to maintain balance despite the impairment to the vestibular system. Through all this, your entire physical being is working harder than it should have to just to operate. Your body and brain respond to the stress they're under, and symptoms like brain fog, memory loss, and fatigue develop. I felt like a thirty-eight-year-old living with dementia. These symptoms were soul-crushing because they were scary! They made my independence feel threatened every day. I feared myself slowly slipping toward complete dependence on others and became worried that my son would be saddled with my care before he was even able to enjoy any of his adulthood and independence. And that was simply not an option. I couldn't fail as a mother now after trying so hard for so long.

I regularly experienced moments of confusion so acute that I struggled with extremely basic tasks. My weekly errands, like self-check-out at the grocery store, were often difficult and perplexing. Completing rote tasks in an orderly fashion —lift the item, scan the item, place it in the bag—was jumbled and discombobulated in my mind. Cooking became a chore. Following even my most familiar family recipes was arduous because the instructions, and the necessary multitasking, I had once completed with ease were now difficult to track (plus the noise naturally associated with working in a kitchen). While out Christmas shopping once, looking to purchase a nice pair of gloves for my mother, I had the incredibly unsettling experience of struggling to put a glove on my hand. I worked at the puzzle like a small child, trying to get each of my five fingers into place but just could not seem to get it right. Finally, I did, but I was stunned, humiliated (despite having no witnesses), and scared. These are moments I will never forget.

I also suffered from derealization while living with SCDS. Derealization is an altered perception of reality, where your environment—surroundings, people, and objects around you—does not appear real. It can feel as though you are outside of yourself watching things happen, or it can feel as though there is some kind of filter between what you are seeing and what is reality. It's like walking around in a dream-like state. This is incredibly frustrating as reality feels just outside of your grasp, and you are aware of it, but you cannot change it. It's like you want to wake up, but you cannot.

SCDS manifests via more commonplace physical symptoms as well. Headaches, fatigue, and heart palpitations, oh my. Headaches were a daily part of life, really throughout my whole life, but most especially during the two years I was living with an active dehiscence. The front right quadrant of my head experienced an almost constant headache, sometimes a dull ache, other times a roaring migraine. I used to say if I could just cut that one quadrant out of my head, I would be completely fine. The fatigue was also overwhelming. I couldn't make it through a workday without at least a short cat nap, and even still, I was in my bed by 6:30 pm virtually every night. I was lucky we were still working from home because of the pandemic; otherwise, I'm not sure if I could have returned to work or would've needed to seek disability. I dragged my body around from task to task, for eight to ten hours per day, then immediately took to my bed to be alone with my SCDS and hibernate. This was my way of surviving. I began experiencing regular heart palpitations; one night, I experienced a heart palpitation so intense it felt like a fish flopping in my chest. My physical wellbeing declined significantly. Exercising felt impossible, not only due to the fatigue but also the fact that my auditory symptoms were deafeningly loud when my heart rate increased, my heartbeat pounding away in my head. A gentler form of exercise, something like yoga, was difficult because bending over would lead to pressure-induced dizziness and/or vertigo. It seemed any attempts at all of living a normal life were thwarted by SCDS.

This was especially salient for me in my work life. My professional accomplishments are some of my proudest and, honestly, as unfortunate as I now understand it to be, at the time, my success at work was inextricably bound to my feelings of self-worth. If I was not *over*achieving at work, I was just another teen mom, a disappointment. At the time, my identity hinged almost entirely on my professional reputation and sense of accomplishment at work. Struggling at work, therefore, represented a much more significant personal battle. SCDS forced me to see this and to do the hard work of separating my worth as a human being from my professional life and from my parenting status. But more on this later.

As I struggled with how to manage my SCDS while working, one decline that really stood out for me was my difficulty with typing and written communication. Two skills that I'm ordinarily very proud of and rely on significantly. While battling SCDS, I consistently used the wrong words. I typed similar, but incorrect, words in almost every sentence. "Talk" instead of "take"; "encouraged" instead of "excited." I sent more than one business email that made little or no sense upon rereading and would then have to follow-up to clarify my initial message. Over time, I established a habit of reading and rereading every report, every email, every work communication four or five times before I would find and correct all my mistakes and call it complete.

My workdays became a prison of repetition. Every task took two or three times longer than it should have. In my two years struggling with SCDS, I made more mistakes at work than I ever made in the fifteen years prior *combined*. Some of these mistakes were significant—to me, anyway. I had fifty-four staff members counting on me every day and a campus full of students whose lives I'm committed to positively impacting. Suddenly, my career, my legitimacy, my identity was fading away. By having such a drastic impact on my professional output, SCDS was making me question everything. *Can I do this job? Can I succeed? Do I deserve this? Can I be a capable leader? Am I letting my team down? What if it gets worse?* My thoughts were an endless parade of self-doubt and worry.

The psychological response to this cognitive decline was unavoidable. The depression and anxiety that so often accompany SCDS were significant for me. I was constantly tearful, brimming with emotion, and socially withdrawn. I had no interest or energy to engage in any non-essential activity. I worried incessantly. I was angry, irritable, and having difficulty being kind to those few people who were trying to support me through this. With SCDS, I struggled mightily not only with my daily symptoms but also the fact that I knew I *looked* totally normal, and yet the symptoms were so unbelievable and bizarre to describe to someone, it was just easier not to tell people what was going on. So, I started hiding myself from the world, literally and figuratively.

SCDS really forced me into an existential crisis. *Who am I? Why am I experiencing this? What is life's purpose? Where do I go from here? Should I consider surgery or try to live my life like this? Can I really go to sleep for four hours while someone drills open my skull, cuts my jaw muscle, and lifts my temporal lobe up so they can attempt to fix the holes in my skull? Holy shit. That is scary to think about! What if it doesn't work? Can I afford to have surgery? Will someone take care of me? Can I really stand the idea that I will likely feel worse before I feel better?* The depths of the fear, the self-questioning, and the isolation truly cannot be described.

All this is not formally acknowledged by the medical community as symptoms of SCDS. But I haven't spoken to anyone with SCDS who doesn't describe these 'other' symptoms. The impact on your life is everywhere. Every day is a grind. Survival is a choice, and I had to wake up every day and choose to survive another day with SCDS...for now.

3

SURVIVAL

"This very moment is the perfect teacher."

– Pema Chödrön

I RELIEF AND TERROR

When the PA called with my CT results, that was a pivotal moment in my life. It was a short but life-changing call. We hung up, and that was that. A wave of peace rolled over me, realizing that the fight for a diagnosis was over.

That peace, though, was intermingled with a feeling of dread quickly creeping to the surface. After speaking with the PA, I found myself alone in my kitchen, standing in stunned silence. I called my mother and cried my eyes out, feeling this odd blend of relief and terror. I wanted to crawl my way out of this dark forest, but the idea of this surgery was so overwhelming. I wanted to be cured of this noisy hell my life had become, but at the same time, I spent hours every day second-guessing myself, wondering if I was even sick at all or if I was making it all up. Living with an invisible illness is unspeakably confusing and frustrating. Even though I finally knew my symptoms were real, I still questioned *how* sick I was, how debilitated I was, and whether there was any part of this that was imagined.

The first few days after the diagnosis were a frenzy of thoughts and questions. I had barely any understanding of SCDS. (Don't forget I diagnosed myself after reading just one article online. And I was still terrified—and I do mean terrified—that someone would tell me I didn't have SCDS). Nonetheless, there was excitement at the diagnosis, and it was two-fold. I knew what was wrong, and I knew it wasn't life-threatening, but I quickly became overwhelmed by how much I needed to know and how little I did know. *What is it I'm living with? How did I get it? Is it permanent? Will it keep getting worse? Does anyone else have it? Is this specialist I'm being referred to any good? What the hell do I do now?* I had no answers—just a diagnosis.

Understanding and pursuing treatment options for SCDS is not easy. This condition has taught me that no matter where you live, regardless of what type of healthcare system your country offers, getting the best medical treatment available is often incredibly difficult.

Six weeks after my CT scan and initial diagnosis, I met the specialist in Boston that my ENT had referred me to. Here was another doctor with a wonderful bedside manner, as kind and attentive as all the other doctors had been. When he entered the room, he introduced himself and launched into an explanation of the surgery he provides for SCDS patients. I interrupted him mid-sentence to ask, "So, you definitely think I have a dehiscence?" He almost laughed while replying, "Oh definitely, yes. There is an obvious dehiscence."

The only diagnosis I had received was over the phone from my original ENT. I was carrying so much anxiety that someone somewhere was going to tell me that's not what I had, and I'd have to start all over hunting for a diagnosis—but he didn't. Instead, he turned his computer monitor to me and showed me my CT scans. He pointed right to the dehiscence so I could see it.

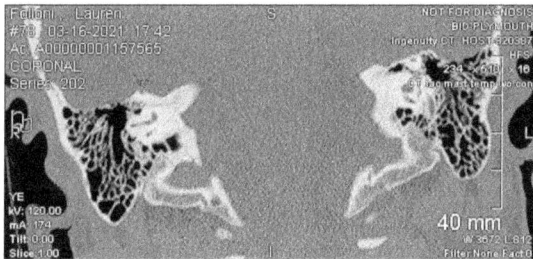

Seeing the dehiscence in my superior canal was such a good feeling. Now I had seen it with my own two eyes! It was real! I was not insane. He took the time to walk me through each and every image of the CT scan and explain what I was looking at. He showed me the difference between my right and left sides so I could clearly see what it should look like since my left ear was healthy. He taught me so much about SCDS during this appointment.

Once I had seen the physical proof of my dehiscence and was able to breathe a sigh of relief, we were able to get back to what he had started to explain about surgery. He explained to me that the surgery he performs is called a Transmastoid Cartilage Cap (TM). He reported that he'd had great success with the TM surgery, and it was the only surgery he did for SCDS.

At this point, my research had taught me that there were three surgeries commonly performed with SCDS patients: Transmastoid Cartilage Cap (TM), Middle Fossa Craniotomy (MFC), and Round Window Reinforcement. The two most common today are the TM and MFC. Which surgery each patient receives seems to depend largely on the doctor they see, but hopefully, it's also based on which approach is best for the patient's individual circumstance.

From my limited understanding of the procedures, they differ in important ways. The TM surgery allows the surgeon to access the inner ear from below without having to perform a craniotomy. This surgery is less invasive than an MFC, but because it approaches from underneath, the surgeon never has a direct view of the dehiscence. The TM is often performed as an outpatient surgery, so patients are released from the hospital the same day. The MFC, on the other hand, is much more involved. This surgery is a craniotomy, meaning the surgeon opens the patient's skull. The MFC involves cutting the jaw muscle, opening the skull, "retracting" the brain's temporal lobe dura (lifting it out of the way, basically) and accessing the inner ear from above. This gives the surgeon direct access to see the dehiscence while they are working. Additionally, there are surgeons performing MFCs that are called "keyhole" MFC. In a keyhole surgery, the surgical opening of the skull is much smaller because the surgeon utilizes an endoscope during the surgery to access the area of the dehiscence. This allows the procedure to be much less invasive. For keyhole MFC patients, that often means less hair shaved, a smaller incision, and possibly faster recovery time. Both surgeries are closed with a titanium plate and screws.

Like everything in life, the surgical options seemed to have long lists of pros and cons that varied from patient to patient. Neither surgery guaranteed its outcomes, and everything I was reading online and discussing with other SCDS patients on Facebook indicated that a patient's SCDS symptoms could actually be worse after a failed surgery. Total and permanent hearing loss in the surgical ear was a risk. Vertigo and/or dizziness would definitely be worse right after surgery and *should* improve over the first year post-surgery but could be a permanent problem. Plus, a host of other potential risks that come from having skull-base surgery: facial paralysis, cerebro-spinal fluid leak, stroke, and meningitis. I had never undergone general anesthesia and had no experience with any major medical treatment. Despite how miserable my life was, I knew things could be worse, and surgery felt like a gamble. I was extremely conflicted about whether or not I should pursue surgery. I knew this was a point in my journey where I would require medical expertise and guidance from the most experienced surgeon I could find.

When I met this first surgeon, I found it interesting that he only performed one of the surgeries. I did not know how doctors decided which surgery they would offer to their patients. Was it personal preference? Was it based on what medical training they had? I had no idea. I just knew he only performed the TM. So, he explained the TM procedure to me in detail and told me that I was a good candidate for the surgery. He then asked if I wanted to have surgery! I nearly fell out of my chair. I felt like he was asking me the most important question of my lifetime, and doing so in such a nonchalant manner, after knowing him for all of fifteen minutes! I had to remind myself this was his job, and it wouldn't be good for anyone if he was as stunned by all this as I was.

This is one of the most difficult things about SCDS. The patient often decides when it's time to have surgery. When you can't live with your symptoms anymore, it's time for surgery. When you are debilitated and can't function, it's time for surgery (but hopefully, you consider it before you reach that point). When the reward outweighs the risks, it's time for surgery. These are very hard judgment calls to make! Especially when you likely spent a long time living with symptoms and wondering if they were even real. I was working so hard to arrive at a place where I truly trusted myself and believed that my symptoms were real, but I wasn't quite there yet—and I knew I needed to be before I even began to *consider* surgery, never mind schedule it.

I told this doctor that I was not ready for surgery yet. I guess I just needed more time to sit with it as an option now that surgery had been officially offered to me, more time to process my options, continue my research, consider the timing as my son was about to start his senior year, and process my fears. He told me that was just fine, scheduled a six-month follow-up appointment for us, and said we'd check in then to see how I was doing. And that was it. I walked out of his office and went home.

Now I had more questions than ever before. I knew I had SCDS. I knew it could get worse over time, but it might not. I knew that surgery was an option, and I knew that one local surgeon believed me to be a good candidate for surgery. So, why didn't I feel better?

Well, for one thing, I was still sick. The term *daily grind* took on a whole new meaning for me. I literally dragged my body around from one place to the next. I was completely empty, exhausted, and distraught most of the time. I also felt really painted into a corner. *What the hell am I supposed to do here? I worked so hard to get here, but where have I really gotten?* I had answers, but I didn't feel like I had any solutions.

At this point, I was thirty-seven years old and had been the picture of health my whole life. I had never had any type of surgery other than wisdom teeth removal. I had never experienced general anesthesia. The thought of having a craniotomy was terrifying. I needed to learn more so that I could arm myself with knowledge. I wasn't ready to accept surgery so easily, and so researching continued to be how I spent all my spare time and my very little spare energy.

For now, I was motivated to avoid surgery as long as possible (because I was *entirely* too afraid of the risks), so figuring out how to survive with SCDS became my primary focus.

II LIVING WITH SCDS

Learning to live with SCDS didn't happen overnight (and I'm not sure I ever fully mastered it), but over time, I spun myself a web of self-care. I tuned into my needs and opened my mind to whatever supports I could gather to survive each day with SCDS.

I was already familiar with the wellness wheel[1] because I use it both personally and professionally. It was created in 1976 by Dr. Bill Hettler who co-founded the National Wellness Institute. Today, it exists in various forms. I use this one from the Substance Abuse and Mental Health Services Administration (SAMHSA)[2] which includes eight dimensions of wellness.

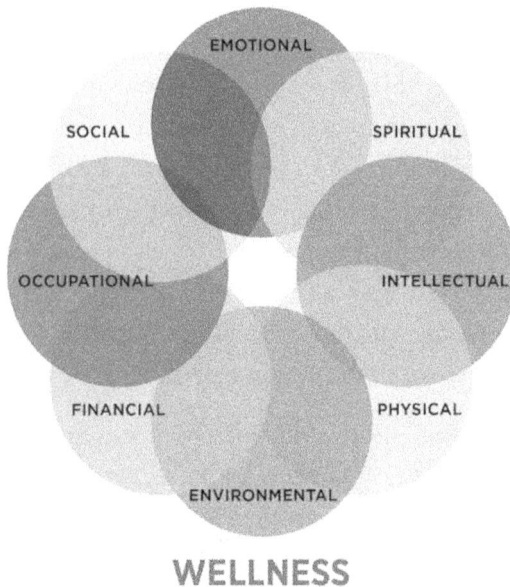

WELLNESS

I began to reflect on each of the eight dimensions of wellness: emotional, spiritual, intellectual, physical, environmental, financial, occupational, and social. I knew if I was going to live with SCDS, I needed to find ways to develop my coping skills in all eight areas.

Surviving with SCDS really does take this level of intentional commitment to taking care of yourself. Life is hard for all of us. We all experience suffering. In the face of the trauma I experienced in my teenage and young adult years, I thought I had mostly figured out how to care for my mental health. I've been in and out of therapy for most of my life. I had deep, lifelong friendships that carried me when I was down. I believed I had overcome every obstacle placed in my path and had come out stronger on the other side. It wasn't until I lost control of my body that I realized how fragile my mental health was and how ineffective most of my go-to coping skills were. Hot showers, comfort food, and pedicures really don't get the job done long-term. They're much too shallow and fleeting. Really meaningful self-care runs much deeper, and SCDS forced me to mine those deepest places inside of me and conjure up a new strength that I never even knew was there.

III EMOTIONAL WELLNESS

I was afraid I was facing a lifelong battle with this invisible condition, and I was tired and frustrated. To this point, I had convinced myself that finding a diagnosis would be the end of the journey, but now I realized it was just the beginning, and that felt like a kick in the teeth. I wanted so badly to scream at the world for making me question myself for so long and for the isolation that was making this journey even harder.

It was clear I needed a lot of emotional support. I was still crying every day, which, in theory, is good because it's one of the body's ways of relieving stress and the feeling of being overwhelmed, but crying made all my SCDS symptoms worse—headaches, head pressure, pulsatile tinnitus, etc.

I felt as fragile as a sandcastle. Just one large wave, one strong gust of wind, and I could crumble into a billion tiny grains of sand, with nothing left of what used to be me. I needed to be propped up by the gentle patting of someone else's hands. I needed a network of people to surround me with love. I didn't feel capable of doing this alone.

I leaned heavily on my usual support system: my mother, my best friends, and my partner at the time. I cried to all of them on many occasions. I talked through all the options, asked their advice, and occasionally yelled at them when my frustration reached a boiling point. These are people who checked in with me on a regular basis to see how I was doing. Most nights, they did my household chores while I tucked myself into bed before 7:00 pm. They listened to me cry and allowed me to be vulnerable. They mailed me cards. They didn't call me crazy when I described my crazy symptoms; *they believed me.* They modified social plans so that I could be in controlled, comfortable environments with tolerable noise levels. They learned about SCDS along with me. They asked me questions and were genuinely interested in my wellbeing. Receiving this love, and feeling this sense of togetherness, kept me afloat on my worst days.

I am incredibly fortunate to have had these amazing people walking this journey with me. I knew I was never alone, but I still felt so lonely trying to survive every day with these wild symptoms. I was desperate to connect with someone else experiencing what I was experiencing.

I recently watched a documentary about Earvin "Magic" Johnson, where he described the early days after he received his HIV diagnosis. He said: "I had to find somebody who is living with the disease who is going to help me understand what my journey is going to be now." His words captured my own feelings perfectly. I had a longing to talk with someone who had walked in my shoes. I was in desperate need of peer support, and through the wonder of social media (you read that right—it's not all bad), I found exactly that. I quickly discovered two private groups to join online. Both groups were formed with the primary purpose of bringing together people suffering with SCDS to provide support to one another and learn from each other.

Each group had 3-4,000 members when I joined (many members in both groups, like I am) from across the world! In an instant, I was transported out of my isolation and into a world full of people just like me. As I scrolled through the posts, reading stories, hearing people describe symptoms identical to mine, all I could do was cry. These people understood me; they weren't just being kind and sympathetic. These people were living the same hell I was. These people were using the same words and phrases to describe their wacky symptoms that I used. It was overwhelming to have this instant connection to, and way to communicate with, people who understood—they really, truly understood! That felt like a miracle.

On top of the sense of belonging I found there, those pages contained a wealth of information. Members had graciously shared many documents and resources with the group to help others understand our condition. There I found a treasure trove of questions to ask doctors, television, and video clips of SCDS patients and doctors describing the condition, and much, much more. I began spending two or three hours every day in these groups—learning, asking questions, and soaking in the idea that I was not completely alone anymore. At the end of each day, I retreated from the physical world into this social media world, where I was surrounded by people like me. I could never thank this wonderful community enough. They are my teachers, healers, friends, confidantes, and heroes. This community of #SCDSwarriors, as we call ourselves, was the antidote to my alienation and gave me a shot of courage and understanding whenever I needed it.

Family and peer support were life savers, but in addition, I needed professional help. I began working with a therapist to talk through what I was experiencing. The impact of this help was immediately apparent. I'm infamous for saying that all humans need therapy, so this was a time when I needed to take my own advice. Therapy is the gift of someone's undivided, unbiased attention. It's an opportunity to share everything on my mind without hearing concern or facing judgment from friends or family. If nothing else, it's an hour of "me time" when I can talk about myself and my thoughts and worries and nothing else. Eventually, I added anxiety medication to my wellness routine because I could think of no reason to make this journey any harder than it had to be.

IV SPIRITUAL WELLNESS

Several years ago, I started studying the basic principles of Buddhism. My curiosity about Buddhism was sparked by two things: my knowledge of mindfulness and meditation as effective coping skills and my personal struggle to figure out how, or if, religion could ever fit into my life again.

Between my own life experiences and my social work training, I have learned a lot about mindfulness. Mindfulness is the ability to stay fully present in the current moment, not reliving the past or worrying about the future. I once had a therapist tell me that when I mastered mindfulness, I would find enjoyment in the simplest tasks, like emptying the dishwasher! I laughed at the time, but now I understand how true that is. When we're able to release ourselves from the past, and put aside anxieties about what the future holds, even for a fleeting second, all we are left with is the experience of this present moment in time, which is a blissful experience when it's occurring without distraction. I recommitted to my mindfulness practice as one way to live with SCDS. I used tools such as the Calm app for guided meditations, the Secular Buddhism podcast for continued learning, and lots of books/articles by top spiritual leaders such as Thich Nhat Hahn and the Dalai Lama.

I had a spiritual void in my life that I was looking to fill. I was raised in the Catholic religion and, even as a kid, was typically happy to go to church on Sundays. The tradition, ceremony, and symbolism central to the religion gave me peace and comfort, a feeling I never got anywhere else in life. I actively practiced Catholicism into adulthood and was raising my son in the Church as well.

In 2002, the same year my son was born, *The Boston Globe* published an article that rocked the world with details of longstanding sexual abuse cover-ups in the Church. This turned out to be just the tip of the iceberg as decades of abuse at the hands of thousands of priests was uncovered. That profound negligence and lack of care, plus the Church's intolerance for so much of humanity—discrimination against the gay community (which includes many of my loved ones), narrow-mindedness toward unwed mothers (which was me!), and an archaic devotion to a patriarchal system, to name a few—forced me to eventually accept (with a little help from my wise son) that this was not a tradition I could continue to devote myself to. I mean, seriously, if I couldn't even be sure that church was a safe environment for my son, how could I continue to participate? I had no choice but to abandon the only religious practice I had ever known.

For close to a decade, I lived a life basically barren of spirituality until I was introduced to the fundamentals of Buddhism by way of mindfulness. Unlike Catholicism, Buddhism gave me a way to practice my own spiritual life by my own rules, without the confines of a strict, authority-driven, fear-based way of life. Buddhism shows us that we are the answers to our own questions and struggles. The peace and comfort we seek are within us already, from birth 'til death. We just need to summon it to the surface. The teachings of the Buddha, called the Dharma, are not something or someone you're asked to believe in, as many religious faiths ask you to believe in a god or deity. Instead, the Dharma teachings are a way of life. They are actions we take.

Buddhism outlines The Four Noble Truths, the first of which is the "truth of suffering," which reminds us that all humans experience suffering. It's just a part of life. There is freedom in acknowledging that we aren't alone when we are suffering. In some way, all humans can relate to our suffering as it's an experience we all share. The teachings of the Dharma can be interpreted in a variety of ways, leaving room for many schools of thought and various approaches to living a life guided by Buddhism. They also teach us to strengthen our ability to endure suffering without adding to it. They teach us the importance of Sangha, or community. The Buddha, the Dharma, and the Sangha—known as The

Three Jewels—were those long-missing puzzles pieces, clicking into place for me and at exactly the right time when I was seeking ways to live with SCDS every day.

I won't lie. It wasn't always easy. Quiet meditation is not always a tranquil experience when your heartbeat is booming in your ear. Dedicating some time each week to reading books or articles is difficult when reading is accompanied by the crunching sound of your eyeballs scrolling across the page and the booming heartbeat in your ear. Really, dedicating time each week to learning anything new was challenging when my life was so marred by brain fog and fatigue. Sleep demanded an exorbitant amount of my time. The most important aspect of increasing the role of Buddhism and mindfulness in my life was to promise myself self-compassion above all else. I wasn't seeking perfection. I was seeking spirituality in whatever small doses were available to me around my SCDS symptoms.

V INTELLECTUAL WELLNESS

I love learning. If I could be a lifelong student and still manage to pay my bills, I would pursue endless education. So, intellectual wellness comes easy to me. I read a lot, and I like to learn new things. Intellectual wellness was an area I didn't have to work that hard on. But, nonetheless, it was a critical part of living with SCDS.

For one thing, I started doing extensive internet research, letting my intuition guide me forward in search of answers to my growing list of questions. It is impossible to live with SCDS without understanding it, and it is impossible to understand it without flexing your intellectual muscles. SCDS is unbelievably complicated, and it's so misunderstood by the medical community it's not something you can just go ask your doctor questions about. There really is no choice but to teach yourself.

But a word of warning: learning about SCDS will produce fear. Fear of the symptoms, fear of living with it, fear of surgery, and so on. It's so important that intellectual wellness is paired with emotional support. That's why the wellness wheel is such a helpful tool. It reminds us that optimal wellness requires work in all eight areas, not just some which could lead to imbalance and actually *increase* stress.

The challenge of intellectual pursuits while living with SCDS is that, honest to God, your brain does. not. work. right. I can't stress enough how prominent those cognitive symptoms described earlier are. Simple things become hard. So, you can imagine how tricky it is to basically put yourself through medical school while you can't remember anything, you can't concentrate, and you have a non-stop headache.

I finished all my degrees before I got sick with SCDS, and I am so grateful for that. I know many SCDS warriors are in school while trying to survive and thrive with this. If you are one of them, my heart goes out to you. You are amazing.

VI PHYSICAL WELLNESS

Oof. This was a hard one. I can't stress enough how important it is to let our bodies guide us without pushing beyond our boundaries. Physical activity while living with SCDS was indescribably difficult for me. I became more sloth than human, spending fifteen or more hours in my bed on an average day. I quickly found that many popular physical activities felt impossible. I enjoyed hiking/walking in the woods, but the pulsatile tinnitus was unbearably loud, a literal bass drum in my ear, and my balance was too unsteady to confidently walk on uneven ground. Yoga and stretching would induce dizziness from bending over. Lifting weights, or even being in a gym, felt beyond reach because the noise of clanking weights was sharp, and I wasn't stable enough on my feet to confidently use cardio equipment.

Walking was the only means of physical activity that felt within my reach. I managed to walk 1-1.5 miles at least four days most weeks, but that was it for physical activity. Even that wasn't easy to manage with the fatigue and the pounding of my footsteps in my ear. With every step, a thump rang out inside my head, and if I pushed myself and elevated my heartrate, my pulsatile tinnitus really would become deafening. My walks were more about trying to maintain some connection to the physical world, to get out of bed and leave the house, than they were about fitness.

A walking routine became even more difficult to maintain after losing my dog and walking partner when he suffered a brief illness and passed away. This is yet another example of the importance of dedicated attention to all eight dimensions of wellness. The grief I experienced after losing my dog significantly impacted my physical wellbeing. It was very difficult to get myself walking again without Booker, the Boston Terrier, trotting ahead of me and stopping to sniff virtually every blade of grass he encountered.

Again, the wellness journey when living with SCDS must start with patience and understanding. I knew from the beginning that all I could do was my best. I didn't want to give up on myself, but I also needed to give myself compassion.

VII ENVIRONMENTAL WELLNESS

Creating an environment conducive to SCDS is one of the first things most SCDS patients seem to do naturally (to avoid tearing your hair out). I was fortunate that I was working from home full-time due to the COVID-19 pandemic at the onset of my SCDS symptoms. This allowed me to have close to full control over my environment. Because my head was a cacophony of internal noises (my voice, my heartbeat, my eyes, my footsteps), I played music and always carried it around with me. This didn't totally drown out the autophony, but it helped take the edge off. It couldn't be too loud, though, because the hyperacusis caused pain in my ears in the face of certain sounds. In the beginning, I made my family remove the TV's surround sound because it was painful. In the end, I only watched TV by myself in my bedroom, where I could set the volume as low as possible.

As described earlier, I also made several other adjustments around the house to ease my pain throughout the day, like switching out dinnerware and cabinet hardware for quieter versions. I completed most household tasks at a snail's pace, both because I was tired and because moving slowly allowed me to control the noise associated with the task at hand, such as putting silverware away as quietly as possible.

Coming up with a sleeping environment was more challenging. I had historically been someone who liked to sleep in pure silence, but SCDS robbed my life of silence. Every night when I lay in bed, I listened to my heartbeat thumping away in my head. I ended up filling the bedroom with overlapping variants of white noise that would distract me from the internal noise but still allow me to sleep—this included a ceiling fan, a floor fan, and the sound of rain. The room was alive with noise, but it was the only way to rest.

VIII FINANCIAL WELLNESS

I'm a recovering workaholic. For much of my life, I worked 80-100 hours per week. Sometimes, that was balancing two jobs, and other times, it was balancing my full-time job with schoolwork. For most of the first year with SCDS, I was working a side job in the evenings as a part-time therapist. This was part of my long-term financial planning, but it didn't take long to figure out I could not continue to work two jobs. I had to let go of the second job to make room for SCDS in my life, which meant I needed to think about alternate ways to pursue or modify my financial goals. Part of that formula meant reconsidering the timelines I had in mind as far as debt reduction and building more savings. In the end, all that really mattered to me was that I was fortunate enough to have stable full-time employment, a desk job that I could stay in while dealing with SCDS. Many SCDS sufferers, such as someone working manual labor or in a very noisy environment, find themselves unable to work. In these situations, financial wellness is a much bigger challenge than it was for me.

My financial priority was understanding what monetary obligations lay ahead for me and preparing for them. I had endless co-pays due to my providers—everything from prescription costs to $20 for every local ENT appointment, to $60 each time I saw a specialist in Boston and $100 for radiology (2 MRIs and a CT scan). Before I was diagnosed with SCDS, I had already spent approximately $600 out of pocket on top of the $600 health insurance premium I was paying *every month*. I saved every receipt from every appointment and every parking garage so that I could claim the deductions on my taxes.

On top of that, I was crunching numbers to determine how I could pursue surgery in another state if I needed to. These exercises led to a moment where my partner and I just looked at each other and said simultaneously, "What if we were poor?!" I was nervous about the long-term costs of my SCDS treatment, but I knew I would be able to get treatment regardless. I also knew that wasn't true for everyone. And my heart ached with the reality that people were out there suffering due to financial barriers to care.

IX OCCUPATIONAL WELLNESS

I know I've made it clear that my professional accomplishments were very meaningful (too meaningful) in my life at the onset of my SCDS. Virtually all the positive feelings I held for myself were wrapped up in my academic and occupational achievements. It was so important for me to be successful in life so that my son could have a mom to be proud of. SCDS plunged me into a situation where I was struggling at work and losing faith in myself as a person. My self-worth was damaged right away and continued to take a beating with every challenge I faced or mistake I made at work, regardless of how trivial they may have seemed to others.

I used several strategies to work toward occupational wellness while I was sick. First, I adjusted my expectations and allowed myself to be human. When I made mistakes, I held myself accountable for them but not prisoner to them! One example is a significant error I made during a historically challenging project, resulting in hundreds of students receiving an email in error. I came completely undone when I realized my mistake and cried, literally, for hours. When I was able to calm down, I picked myself up off the ground (where I sat crying) and finished the project to the best of my ability. I did not continue to beat myself up or stay stuck in the emotion and disappointment of that moment. When it was complete, I reminded myself that, in the end, a very challenging project was now complete, and the error I made couldn't be reversed but could easily be explained and did not have any lasting negative impact.

Part of the way through my SCDS journey, when I was still searching for a diagnosis, I decided to tell my closest coworkers what I was going through. Not only did this provide some explanation for the parade of appointments I found myself going to, but allowing people into my experience, especially those who were most likely to notice a difference in me, helped me to maintain a sense of well-being and balance at work. This is a personal choice, and I know not everyone will choose to disclose something so personal to work colleagues, but for me, it helped me to accept it myself.

Last, but maybe most important, I formally advocated to have my needs met at work. When we returned to working in the office, I pursued medical accommodations with my employer to allow me to continue working most of my work week at home. This was important to my success because, as I mentioned above, I could control my home environ-ment and ease my SCDS symptoms that way.

The positive outcome for me here was that I achieved a realistic definition of occupational wellness for the first time in my life, thanks to SCDS. My occupation is not an indicator of whether I am worthy of love or acceptance as a person. If SCDS hadn't forced me to deal with these demons as I struggled at work, I don't know how long it might have taken me to put work in its rightful place in my life—it's one piece of the pie, not the whole thing.

X SOCIAL WELLNESS

One thing I can guarantee is that SCDS is likely to hamper your social life. Again, I was fortunate that I was mostly sick through the height of the pandemic, so pretty much no one had a social life. There were no parties to attend, and movie theaters and restaurants were closed. Social living was on pause. By this time, my relationship was dissolving quickly, and we were living more as roommates than part-ners. Still, he definitely had to pick up a larger share of the housework since I was mostly in bed when I wasn't working.

When mankind started crawling out of its collective cave, though, and social outings came a-calling, I had to develop a plan for social wellness while living with SCDS. I wanted to act as "normal" as possible, so I took to my social media groups in search of advice for how to venture out into the world. Most people recommended using ear plugs in noisy places, like restaurants. I bought some cheap ear plugs on Amazon and made sure they were always in my purse. I was surprised by how much they helped me to deal with environmental noise, especially in places full of sharp noises like restaurants. They also helped me lessen motion sickness and dizziness when riding in cars. The only drawback was that using an ear plug in my affected ear amplified my internal sounds. But that was the only way to handle an environment full of noise.

It was important for me to accept that I had some limitations while living with SCDS. Just like I couldn't participate in some physical activities, I could not engage in some social activities. Going to the movies was one example. I completely stopped going to movies because it was too painful, and concerts weren't an option either. I had to be willing to set those boundaries with my friends and family without feeling guilty. Taking care of myself was most important. The only social engagements I really committed to were my son's senior year activities. When it came to him, I did my very best to always be present and look as well as I could.

At the same time, this was a time to consider creative solutions for maintaining social connections. Staying in touch with friends via video calls was one excellent way we were able to stay in touch, and I was able to stay at home in my comfortable environment. During this time, my grandmother started calling me regularly on the phone. Ordinarily, I hate talking on the phone (even before SCDS), but I found it was nice to have someone to talk to and to feel less alone during our phone calls. Instead of holding my phone up to my ear, I would use speaker phone, and this was an easy solution as well as an easy way to avoid complete isolation.

I already described the comfort and community I found in the SCDS social media groups, but I need to mention that group again here. This virtual community I joined was my greatest social outlet through SCDS. Not just because I could interact with them from my own home, but also because these were the only people on the planet who could truly understand me. I had a lot of love and support that I was grateful for, but I can't express how meaningful it was to have a conversation with someone who had experienced the same thing as me. It's a social connection that can't be replicated.

This community of support gave me the strength I needed to continue educating myself on this condition and decide my path forward. SCDS was solidifying so many of these wellness skills for me. Only I could decide what happened next; before I could decide, I needed to create the right conditions to make such important decisions.

4

TREATMENT

"I am no bird; and no net ensnares me;
I am a free human being with an independent will"
— Charlotte Brontë, Jane Eyre

I STUMBLING UPON AN EXPERT

While I was researching the complexity of SCDS treatment and surgery, it became clear how important it was to see a doctor with a very thorough understanding of the condition and its treatment options—and it was obvious that there aren't many of them! As an example, I noticed several small spots in my CT scan that looked like holes. I knew they weren't the dehiscence, though, because I had marked that location when the doctor showed it to me. I was puzzled by this but assumed it must be nothing since he hadn't mentioned it when we were reviewing my scans together.

Soon after, I learned about tegmen defects from my social media groups. Tegmen defects are holes in the roof of the middle ear—and I later learned I had several of them. Tegmen defects probably didn't contribute to the symptoms I was experiencing, but they were a problem that needed to be addressed as the brain can sometimes herniate down through those holes and cause major problems. My tegmen defects were never mentioned by the first surgeon, though. I never saw that doctor again, so I don't know whether he would have addressed those if he had performed surgery. My point is that I don't believe I left that appointment fully informed even though the surgeon had offered to immediately take steps toward scheduling surgery for me.

The online groups were filled with stories like mine. Doctors that didn't listen to patients, told them nothing was wrong with them, didn't share all the details with them, or didn't know enough to be helpful. I fully acknowledge that it's no easy feat to understand exactly how the inner ear and vestibular systems work, so we can't expect all doctors to know everything—but is it too much to expect a doctor to listen to their patients, believe them, and research the reported symptoms? Reading all the frustrating stories told by SCDS patients enlightened me to the importance of self-advocacy and seeing doctors as partners in health, *not* authority figures. I learned through this process that a doctor's role is not to tell me what's best for me. Only I can do that (after gathering all the available information, including the medical expertise of a trusted doctor).

That's not to say that the first doctor I met in Boston wasn't a great doctor. I have no reason to believe he isn't. However, in my mind, I was referred to him for business reasons, not medical reasons; he is affiliated with the same hospital that my ENT's office is affiliated with. This really bothered me as I felt like my medical decisions weren't made based on my needs as a patient. I was already so disappointed that my ENT's office had not found the diagnosis, I wasn't willing to accept a specialist's referral based solely on hospital affiliation. So, I set out to figure out options on my own to ensure that I was seeing the best provider for me, not the best business arrangement for hospital administrators.

In these online groups, I read a lot of sad and scary experiences with SCDS, but I also read stories of hope and healing. Many members posted about their surgery experiences, talked about getting their lives back, and living without SCDS post-surgery. I quickly noticed that there were two specific medical teams being discussed *constantly* as some of the best SCDS doctors in the United States, if not the world. I decided I would need to see one of them if I were to pursue surgery someday. However, both were located outside of my home state, and I had no idea if health insurance would cover that. So now I had to start the third leg of my journey and become a health insurance expert, on top of being an expert of my own symptoms and SCDS itself. Every waking moment in my life was dedicated either to my full-time job or SCDS. I was sick and tired. Literally.

After a couple of months of research, I noticed a third doctor's name was regularly circulated in my social media groups, and always—and I do mean *always*—with overwhelmingly positive comments from his patients. Dr. Daniel Lee is an Otologist/Neurotologist at Mass Eye and Ear Infirmary in Boston where he has an "international referral center for the diagnosis and management of superior canal dehiscence syndrome."[1] Thanks to this amazing

LAUREN FOLLONI

social media group, I found out that there was an international expert practically in my own back yard, right here in Massachusetts, that I otherwise would not have known about. It was infuriating to think about being so close to an SCDS expert but not being referred to him by my own ENT.

Anyway, I decided immediately that I had to see him! I was anxious for the opportunity to get a second opinion and also to sit with a doctor with the level of SCDS expertise that Dr. Lee appeared to have. Of course, I immediately discovered that my health insurance didn't cover Dr. Lee, so I was forced to wait several weeks, then change my health insurance provider with my employer (almost doubling my monthly insurance payments), then wait several more weeks for my insurance to change. Only then could I see Dr. Lee.

The frustration from dealing with insurance red-tape, the financial commitment, and *allllll* the waiting felt almost unbearable. In these moments, though, I would try to remind myself how lucky I was. I had only been sick for a year and a half when I found Dr. Lee, while many SCDS patients suffer for years, if not decades or a lifetime. I was financially stable, so I could afford the additional financial commitment to change my health insurance to a plan that covered Dr. Lee. Last, and most importantly, I could drive to Dr. Lee's office in about an hour while many patients are flying across state or international borders to receive care from an SCDS expert. So, while my SCDS journey was difficult to endure (there's no such thing as an easy one), I was much better off than many of my contemporaries, and I tried to remain as grateful as I could.

While I waited for my appointment with Dr. Lee to roll around, I absorbed as much SCDS knowledge as I could to be prepared. I couldn't stand the idea of another disappointment. I spent thousands of hours learning about SCDS—reading websites and research articles, keeping a daily journal of my symptoms, watching video clips of SCDS warriors telling their stories, and asking endless questions in my social media groups. I even watched medical school lectures by the leading SCDS experts! I was going to make sure I was fully prepared to advocate for myself when I met Dr. Lee. I would be strong and unstoppable! I was going to get the care I believed I deserved.

II *CHOOSING* MEDICAL CARE

I would never relinquish my knowledge of SCDS. I'm glad I spent so many hours learning everything I could take in about the condition. It has served me very well through this journey. But it was also immediately clear upon meeting Dr. Lee that it was probably unnecessary (except, of course, that that's what helped me find him). Right away the experience with Dr. Lee was completely different from any other appointment I'd had so far. He was kind, attentive, matter of fact, and straight to the point as the other doctors had been, but he was also very patient in listening to my questions (I always bring a lot), very thorough in his explanations, and spoke with a knowledge of SCDS that I hadn't heard before. He made me feel so calm. In his presence was the first time I felt anything other than terror about my future with SCDS. He explained to me how SCDS was diagnosed through a variety of tests. He answered all my questions. And he introduced me to the tuning fork test.

I don't completely understand how this works, but when a doctor strikes a tuning fork to make it vibrate, and then holds it to your forehead, it's one way to confirm the results of the hearing test. Conductive hyperacusis is the term used to describe the fact that SCDS patients can hear their internal noises. So, when Dr. Lee held that tuning fork to my forehead, an alarm-type of noise started screaming out in my right ear and the whole room went sideways! I was stunned (and a little nauseous)! I had battled eighteen months for a diagnosis, and he seemed to just boil it all down to a momentary test with a tuning fork. Obviously, I know diagnosing SCDS takes much more than a tuning fork, but this appointment really blew my mind in every imaginable way. Later, I remembered that the first surgeon I met also did the tuning fork test, but it was only barely a noise in my right ear at that time, so the memory didn't stick with me the way it always would after this first time Dr. Lee did the tuning fork test. This was yet another sign my SCDS symptoms were likely worsening (or something didn't go right in that first appointment), and I couldn't ignore that.

As we concluded this first meeting, Dr. Lee broached the topic of surgery, saying he believed I was probably a good candidate. He explained that he performs both the TM and MFC surgeries, but that he would opt for the MFC with me. This was because of the location of my dehiscence and that the MFC could give him a full view of it. He also confirmed that I had tegmen defects (those were other holes I thought I saw in my CT scans). He said those holes would be important to correct as well, and he would automatically do that as part of the MFC procedure. Before any additional surgery steps were taken, Dr. Lee first wanted to complete a comprehensive suite of tests to confirm the SCDS diagnosis. He explained to me that that there are at least three tests that doctors give patients with a suspected dehiscence: a CT scan, an audiogram (hearing test), and a VEMP test.

Prior to my appointment, my ENT's office had sent my audiogram results to Dr. Lee, and I *thought* they had sent my CT and MRI scans as well. Turns out they didn't, so I had to start all over with that request, but Dr. Lee was willing to look at the photos I had on my cell phone of my CT scan. Using that, he confirmed that I appeared to have a classic dehiscence of the superior semicircular canal at the location of the arcuate eminence. This just means the hole is at the top of my superior semicircular canal, which is the most common place for a dehiscence to appear.

My CT scan was, of course, already done. Luckily, Dr. Lee said I would not have to have another one. My local ENT's office was aware that CT scans looking for a dehiscence needed to be ordered in a very specific manner. The scan needed to be a high-resolution and thin slice scan (.6mm or less). If I understand correctly, this means the image quality will be sharper, and images would be taken closer together than normal, both important since we're looking for a tiny hole in a tiny bone. I imagine that getting an image of it is not easy.

You might recall that the first test I was ever given in my quest for a diagnosis was a hearing test, and the results came back normal. So, while I had already done a hearing test with my local ENT's office, Dr. Lee ordered another one at Mass Eye and Ear. He explained that many ENT offices don't measure if a patient can hear sounds below zero decibels. Sound does exist below zero decibels, but the average human ear can't hear it. Many SCDS patients, including me, *can* hear it though (listen, we're not joking when we can say that our head is constantly full of noise, and it is exhausting!)—so hearing below that zero threshold is a hallmark sign of a dehiscence. At the end of my hearing test at Mass Eye and Ear, I asked the audiologist what she thought, and she quickly responded that my results did appear to suggest SCDS.

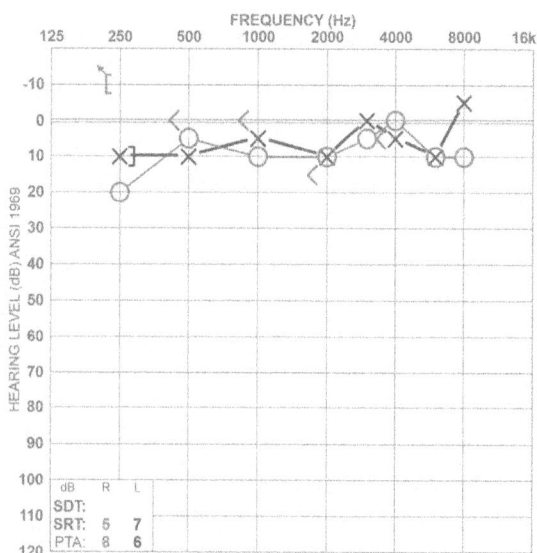

(Quick rant: Why, oh, why does the national standard for audiology exclude measuring for hearing below zero deci-bels in hearing tests?! Think of the positive impact just that simple change in the testing could have on the lives of SCDS patients who are suffering and having such difficulty getting the right diagnosis! I'll never be able to make sense of it).

The third test that SCDS patients will undergo is called a VEMP test. VEMP stands for Vestibular Evoked Myogenic Potentials. I can't pretend to understand the VEMP test. I have probably spent close to 100 hours researching how this test works, and how to read the results, but I still don't fully understand it. What I do know is that there are two kinds: the cervical VEMP (cVEMP) and the ocular VEMP (oVEMP). Both tests place electrodes on the patient (on the neck for cVEMP; under the eyes for oVEMP), then require the patient to basically flex the muscle where the electrode is located. Then, a sound is played for the patient while the muscle is flexed. This test measures how these tiny muscles respond to sound, which gives the doctor information about whether the vestibular system is working as expected.

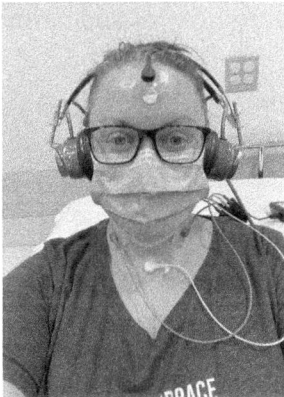

At the end of my cVEMP test at Mass Eye and Ear, I did the same thing and asked the doctor administering the test what she thought. She was careful to say that interpreting VEMP results took some time but that what she was seeing did seem to suggest that I had SCDS.

Next up was my second appointment with Dr. Lee to review all these test results with him, but I had to wait almost two months for that appointment. I was on pins and needles waiting for it. My physical and psychological states had declined significantly over the last several months, and I was now at a point where I wanted to seriously talk surgery with him. I realized that my SCDS symptoms would continue to worsen over time, and I had a hard time imagining how much worse it could possibly get. I had become a shell of a person. I only functioned well enough to get through my workday each day and then go directly to bed. There was very little light left in my life. I reached a point so low that I had to remind myself of that promise I made to myself several months ago, a promise to take care of my body and not ask it to be sick any longer than it had to be. My intuition was guiding me forward. I just needed to work through the fear and guide myself to the other side of this.

I felt safe and secure under Dr. Lee's care. Also, I was on the younger side of the SCDS community—with the average age of diagnosis being 45—and I thought that pursuing major surgery would make sense while I was as young as possible. Also, I had no idea how old Dr. Lee was, but I didn't want to risk his eventual retirement and having to find a different surgeon. The puzzle pieces seemed to be coming together on their own. I knew I would have to climb the unbelievable heights of my fear, and I felt capable of attempting to do that under Dr. Lee's care. I had been relying heavily on my intuition to care for myself through this so far, and it had not failed me yet.

This moment in my SCDS journey is crucial. It's when I *chose* my medical care instead of allowing it to be dictated for me. I found Dr. Lee on my own, and I pursued the necessary health insurance changes to make my choice of provider a reality. I committed to whatever research, whatever waiting, and whatever financial commitments, would be necessary because what was most important to me was my ability to take my care into my own hands. Seeing a doctor based only on the fact that another doctor had referred me to them was not the approach I was willing to take. It was up to me to choose my own path to medical care and when.

What stands out to me about these early experiences at Mass Eye and Ear is that suddenly, *everyone* was telling me I had SCDS! After eighteen long months of searching for answers, now every healthcare provider I encountered was diagnosing me in under an hour! There was a sense of freedom in these conversations. I had been doubting myself and questioning my own symptoms for a very long time. Now all these people were telling me they could provide proof! I used to just sit and stare at my test results, trying to wrap my mind around the fact that all my problems were visible there, right in those test results and scans. The problem, I realized, was not that SCDS is impossible to diagnose. The problem is that general practitioners just do not know enough about it or how to test for it. *How can we connect these dots? How can general practitioners increase their knowledge to the point where they don't have to become experts themselves, but they can quickly determine when an expert is needed and know which expert(s) to refer those patients to immediately?*

SCDS treatment saves lives. And I don't just mean in the figurative way that it saved mine. I did go from being unable to live a normal life at all to being a fully functional person again, but I also mean very literally that proper SCDS treatment saves lives. The despair associated with SCDS symptoms plus inadequate medical care can't be understated. We know that SCDS warriors lose their lives to suicide—and that's an unacceptable fate for our SCDS community, knowing that excellent treatment is out there.

If you are suffering with SCDS-like symptoms and experiencing thoughts of suicide, please seek help. See Appendix

A in this book for a list of resources of people and places who want to listen and help.

III ROLLER COASTER

A very long two months later, it was my turn to see Dr. Lee again. I knew I had completed the three major tests and that we would review the results together in this appointment. I hoped we would also discuss moving toward surgery as soon as possible. Unfortunately, as is so common with SCDS journeys, that didn't go as planned.

I left this appointment feeling defeated and afraid. Dr. Lee explained my VEMP test results, indicating that the right side did show signs of a dehiscence. However, he also said the left side results were abnormal, not indicative of a dehiscence since I had no symptoms on my left side, but in case something *else* was wrong with my left side functioning, he was sending me for a battery of vestibular tests. Dr. Lee explained that more vestibular testing would be necessary before he cleared me for MFC surgery because it was important that my body could rely on a healthy left ear for healing and recovery after my right ear had been operated on.

As sad and scared as I was that this additional testing might mean surgery was no longer an option for me for me at all, I was also grateful for how thorough Dr. Lee was being. Considering how many surgery-gone-wrong stories existed in the social media groups, nothing was more important to me than making sure I had a chance at full recovery if I did pursue surgery. Surgery could make things worse! It's not a decision to be taken lightly. So, while being asked to wait even more, and go through even more testing, felt like asking too much, it was a pill I was willing to swallow.

Three days later, I returned to Mass Eye and Ear to complete the vestibular testing. This series of tests was really difficult. Just being honest. You must stop taking most medications a couple of days before these tests, can't have any makeup or lotions on your face that day, and definitely need a friend or family member there with you to drive home. My mom drove me to this appointment and waited patiently while I endured several different tests. I had to do all these tests without my glasses on, which made it that much harder as I have terrible vision.

The first test was balance testing, which involved getting hooked into a harness that was connected to the ceiling (or something way above my head, anyway). The test required me to walk on a surface that moved unpredictably beneath my feet and try not to fall over or touch the walls to hold myself up. Then, I moved on to a head impulse test, where the technician put their hands on either side of my head, positioned my head correctly, then moved my head side to side slowly at first, then suddenly a very fast movement. This was looking for nystagmus, which is involuntary eye movement in response to sound or motion.

And they saved the best (read: worst) for last, which is videonystagmography (VNG) and caloric testing. I promised myself I'd be honest with you through this entire book, so here goes: this testing was brutal! VNG testing involves wearing goggles that have a camera in them to record your eye movement. You sit in a chair in a dark room and watch images move across the wall in front of you. Even if you have a healthy vestibular system, this is likely to induce vertigo, and the whole room will feel like it's in motion. The roller coaster lovers among us might actually enjoy it!

The main event, though, was the caloric testing. During caloric testing, they put hot and cold water or air into your ear. Sounds innocent enough, but trust me, it isn't. Still wearing the goggles, the technician laid the chair back, so I was almost flat. He then started flushing my ear with water for what felt like an eternity. Almost immediately, hell broke loose, and I experienced a vertigo feeling much more intense than anything I'd ever felt before. It truly felt like I was in full motion, spinning head over feet. Then the technician stopped the water in my ear, and while my vestibular system tried to figure out what the hell was happening, my eyes started darting back and forth unbelievably fast. So this was nystagmus! I was stupefied. I couldn't imagine living with eye movement like this that was completely out of my control, yet many SCDS warriors have to live with this resulting from normal daily tasks, such as certain movements while emptying the dishwasher or weather fluctuations. While my vestibular system was freaking out and trying to regain its composure, the technician asked very basic questions—I guess to keep me distracted? Anyway, he asked me to name a boy's name that starts with an "A," and I could not come up with an answer, even though my son's name begins with A! My brain was complete mush. It was the most intense physical sensation I think I've ever felt. And that was just the first ear.

After the caloric testing torture was over, I was able to go home. The technician had to help me walk down the hall to the locker where my personal items were stored. He also had to unlock the locker because I was still in such a dizzy stupor there was no way I could muster up the fine motor skills necessary to insert a key into a lock. He helped me out to the waiting area, where I found my mother, who immediately asked if I was okay. I told her I was fine, just felt a little drunk and wanted to go. Honestly, I wanted to run as far from that caloric testing as I could! We had a long walk to the elevator, though, and I almost immediately regretted leaving so soon. I couldn't even think enough to realize I needed to sit down for a while before heading into an elevator and out onto the streets of Boston. Within a couple of hours, I felt normal again, but this was a long day, and I was even more committed to pursuing surgery after experiencing that kind of dizziness and vertigo. I would do whatever I could to stop my SCDS from progressing further. I hoped with everything I had that I had passed those vestibular tests and would get Dr. Lee's clearance for surgery when I saw him next. So, now more waiting. My appointment with Dr. Lee was a little over a month away.

The month dragged—I mean, it *really* dragged. During this time, it was becoming increasingly clear that my relationship was nearing its end. As I prepared to see Dr. Lee again, I was also preparing for going through surgery and recovery as a single person. I knew I had the strength of my family and friends to draw from, so I focused on my health as we began to transition out of our relationship. Finally, the day I had been waiting for arrived, and I headed into Boston for my fifth visit to Mass Eye and Ear in as many months. This appointment happened to fall on my son's nineteenth birthday. I was hoping this coincidence would give me some much-needed luck. And maybe it did—because on November 18, 2021, Dr. Lee cleared me for right-side keyhole Middle Fossa Craniotomy (MFC)!

He reviewed all the surgery details with me again, reminding me that surgery is the only treatment option available for SCDS, and MFC is major surgery with several risks to consider. He reassured me that his experience with SCDS patients was extensive, with very few complications after surgery. He talked me through what to expect during recovery. I should plan to be out of work for at least four weeks (with most people I knew online staying home from work for more like eight weeks). I would be in the hospital for two or three nights, with the first night in the intensive care unit (ICU), which is the normal procedure after this surgery as they monitor you closely through that first night. Dr. Lee shared that I would likely have a physical therapy session before being released from the hospital and that I should expect to be off-balance in the weeks following surgery. Many patients use a cane for a while, and some require vestibular therapy to help regain balance. He also reminded me that in order to access the inner ear during surgery, the jaw muscle would be cut. As a result, associated pain should be expected during recovery. Patients usually opt for soft foods, small/soft bristle toothbrushes, etc., as opening your mouth wide is difficult in the beginning.

In the end, I knew I was facing a decision to live this painful life or to put my trust in Dr. Lee and pursue my only treatment option. It was Dr. Lee's thorough evaluation of me before clearing me for surgery, his dedication to selecting the surgical procedure that was best for my specific case of SCDS, and his willingness to answer my questions and share his expertise and knowledge with me that gave me the confidence to commit. I told Dr. Lee I was ready—my exact words might have been, "Let's do this!"

Dr. Lee told me that he was scheduling surgeries into February 2022 at that point and that I could expect a phone call the following week to schedule my surgery date! Then I signed the surgery waiver with him, and he sent me on my way. All that was left now was (even more) waiting. This time, for surgery.

IV WAITING

I waited through fall and winter for my surgery date to eventually come around. These were long, dark New England months, both literally and figuratively. The unstable weather patterns of winter made all my symptoms worse, so daily life was harder, days were shorter, and my anxiety was much higher. Despite the challenges, I had several priorities to address while I waited for surgery; they mostly centered again around that wellness wheel, making sure that I was as mentally, physically, financially, and spiritually prepared as I could be.

I am a planner by nature, a list-maker. My life was full of lists as I prepared for my MFC. I had a list of questions for the doctor, a list of questions for my peers on social media, a list of recovery supplies to buy, a list of health insurance questions and tasks, and a list of work tasks to complete. I even had a list of movies and TV shows to watch while I was recuperating. Were all these lists necessary? Probably not, but they helped me manage my anxiety, which was priceless.

I was having nightmares regularly about surgery-gone-wrong scenarios. I struggled to get any quality sleep at all, even though so much of my time was spent in bed. I was having major difficulty in my interpersonal relationships. I was isolating to an extreme, pushing away loved ones, and becoming angry when they tried to offer support.

This was when I started taking anxiety medication. I didn't want to let my fears negatively affect my relationships with the people who had been so supportive of me, my mom especially. I think many of us are guilty of being especially open (read: mean) to our mothers because we know their love is unconditional. I didn't want my suffering to create suffering for her, though, as I grew more and more intolerable. I was also becoming concerned that I would cancel my surgery out of fear. I knew I needed to address the overwhelming anxiety. So, I had an appointment with my primary care doctor to discuss the possibility of medication. She gave me an anxiety assessment, and I scored something like an eighteen out of twenty! The next day, I filled a Prozac prescription and called Dr. Lee's office to ensure it was okay to begin a new medication shortly before surgery. Over the next few weeks, I slowly started to feel a little better so that I could at least handle my daily stressors and symptoms without the added crippling anxiety about surgery.

I tried to identify ways that I could use this waiting time productively to set myself up for recovery success after surgery. I recommitted to being as physically active as possible without pushing myself too hard. I tried to walk one mile every day in the months leading up to surgery. When it was bad weather, I did it inside using walking videos online.

I researched all my options for medical leave at work. In the end, I was incredibly fortunate to be able to take ten weeks medical leave from work using the Family Medical

Leave Act (FMLA) and my earned sick time. As a long-time state employee of the Commonwealth of Massachusetts, I was fortunate to have accumulated enough sick time to cover this leave with no impact on my income. This allowed me to take the time I knew I would need to fully recover without the pressure of rushing back to my busy and fast-paced job before I was ready. Others have pursued creative solutions to create the necessary recovery time in their lives, such as using disability benefits.

I also tried to find ways to comfort myself during this time of high anxiety. Like so many in my generation, I grew up loving Disney movies. For several weeks in a row leading up to my surgery, I watched a Disney movie every night. It was a simple way to recall the comfort of childhood and self-sooth as I mentally prepared for what I believed was going to be the fight of my life to get through this surgery and be healed from SCDS.

5

HEALING

"All that we are arises with our thoughts.
With our thoughts we make the world."
— *The Buddha*

I SURGERY

On March 18, 2022, exactly four months after Dr. Lee cleared me for surgery, my mother and I awoke in a Boston hotel room. We stayed there the night before so we wouldn't have to drive into Boston the morning of (if you're at all familiar with Boston traffic, I know you get this). My mother would stay in the hotel the first night after my surgery as well so she could remain near the hospital.

Shortly after waking up, we walked the quarter mile over to Mass Eye and Ear for my MFC. My surgery was scheduled for 10:45 am and we were told to arrive by 8:30 am to ensure plenty of time for the check-in and preparation procedures. I felt nervous that morning but also excited. At that point,

I just wanted it to be over. I was so afraid the surgery would not succeed or my recovery would be long and painful, but there was only one way to find out.

Once at the hospital, we waited for maybe a half-hour before a nurse came to get me. I went alone with her to a big room full of patients awaiting a variety of different surgeries (separated by curtains) and staff. She and I talked briefly to review my medical history, etc. Then she sent me back to the waiting room with my mother. A little while later, probably around 10:00 am, I was called back again to that big room, this time to begin my pre-operative care. My mother was able to come with me and stay until I was taken away to the operating room (OR).

We spent a long time in this room together, around two hours. This is when I changed into a hospital gown and was hooked up to IVs to start certain IV medications before surgery. This is also when I received a Scopolamine patch, which is an anti-nausea patch. This was very important to me because I was constantly reading stories on social media of people being very dizzy and having nausea and vomiting throughout their first night after surgery. I just knew I needed to do whatever I could to avoid that happening to me, so it was important to me to request the patch.

Also, during this time, a parade of medical staff came to see me. This is when I met the anesthesiologists, the OR nurse, a medical fellow who would be observing my surgery, and several more people; there were so many people coming and going, I honestly can't remember who they all were.

I know I saw Dr. Lee, though. My nerves practically melted away when he came to see me and, with his steady, calm presence, assured me everything was going to be fine. Dr.

Lee marked the ear that would be operated on. He also introduced his two colleagues for the first time: Dr. Yohan Song and Dr. Lauren Miller. Dr. Song and Dr. Miller are important here because they are the doctors who attended to me during my hospital stay after the surgery. I saw Dr. Lee once after my surgery, that evening several hours after my surgery was complete. After that, I didn't see him again until my two-week follow-up appointment, where I would have my stitches removed. That was just fine by me. Dr. Song, Dr. Miller, and the entire nursing staff were very attentive and caring. I felt very well cared for the entire time I was in the hospital.

By the time I finally went into surgery, it was after noon, so my procedure started close to two hours after it was scheduled to begin. However, it was also much shorter than I was expecting it to be—at least, that's what they told me. My last memory is being wheeled into the OR and moving myself on to the operating table. Then they immediately put an oxygen mask on my face, and that's the last thing I recall. Approximately two hours later, my surgery was done, and my mother received a phone call saying that I was out of surgery, and she could come back to the hospital to see Dr. Lee (she had opted to wait in the hotel room while I was in surgery). Dr. Lee met with her briefly to explain the surgery and said everything went well. He gave her several photos that were taken during the operation and told her my dehiscence ended up being smaller than average.

My dehiscence was 2 millimeters long. That's about the size of the tip of a sharp crayon! It's mind-boggling to think of such a tiny hole ripping through my life like a tornado. When we remember that the entire vestibular system is the size of a quarter, though, it helps to maintain perspective.

These systems are incredibly tiny but, at the same time, so vital to our health and wellbeing.

I remember waking up in the post-op room, which was just like the room I was in before surgery (maybe it was the same room? I really don't know). When I woke up, there was a nurse sitting beside me. She introduced herself to me. I know that because I remember her name was Amy. She checked on my vitals, etc., and then a couple of people brought me to have a CT scan done, which I have virtually no memory of. From there, I was brought up to the ICU where I would spend my first night. I don't remember much of the first night, aside from the people.

I made it to the ICU room around 5:30 pm. A nurse named Andrea was with me throughout my first night. She was wonderfully kind and caring. She made me feel very comfortable and cared for. Compared to what I was expecting, I had very little pain this first night. That first night, I rated the pain as a 7 on a scale of 10, but I remember that was headache pain. I didn't have much pain associated with the incision itself. At this point, and through my entire hospital stay, I was wearing the head dressing to cover the incision.

I didn't have any nausea at all, thanks to the patch. I did have severe vertigo and dizziness for the first twenty-four hours or so. I couldn't move at all without the room spinning. I was still catheterized for this first night, so I wasn't very mobile anyway. I did my best to stay still and rest.

Not too long after I was settled into the ICU room, my son and my sister came to visit me. It was so nice to see their familiar faces and hold their hands for a while. I don't remember much of my time

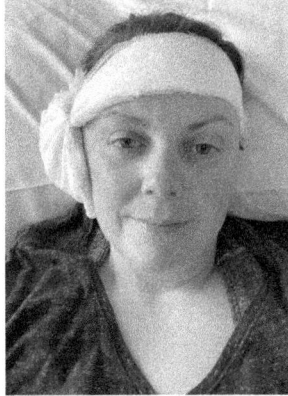

with them, or how long they stayed, but I know I was very emotional and cried. I suspect that was more from the meds than anything else. I wasn't sad or upset, though I was feeling apprehensive about spending the night in the hospital alone. I never did feel alone, though, because Andrea was checking on me so often, and I was still pretty loopy from the meds. Due to COVID restrictions in the hospital, I could only have two visitors per day, so my sister-in-law and mother were in the waiting room while my son and sister visited with me. I asked to video call them, so we were able to do that and see each other quickly. That was nice because it was hard not being able to see all my loved ones in person right away after surgery.

Dr. Lee happened to visit while my son and sister were with me. He didn't stay long, and the only things I can remember about his visit are that I was *so* happy to see him and hear him say everything went well and that he used something to scratch on the head dressing and see if I could hear it. This happened each time a doctor visited me in the hospital. Dr. Lee explained it was part of their standard practice to get an early sense of whether there was any hearing loss resulting from the surgery. I was happy to report that I could hear the scratching. Also, this was the first time I noticed that I could not hear my eyes moving or my heart beating! I knew it was way too early to know the surgery results, but it certainly seemed like my surgery was a success so far!

My family visited with me for a while longer after Dr. Lee left. They made sure I had my personal belongings, most importantly my cell phone and ear buds so I could listen to music. There was no TV in the room. This ICU room seemed large enough to have four patients in it with curtain dividers, but for this night, there were two of us. The other patient was an older woman who was experiencing great discomfort throughout the night. I was grateful for my music and the amazing nurses who took such great care of my roommate and me all night long. I remember feeling hot through the night, which wasn't helping my headache. At one point, Andrea brought me an ice pack, which I kept on my forehead. That was great.

The next morning, my catheter was removed and, a while later, they brought me breakfast, which I was able to eat with no problem. My agenda for the day included trying to walk around a bit, going for an MRI, a visit from a physical therapist, and hopefully moving out of the ICU room. I was feeling dizzy and unsteady on my feet, but the vertigo was a lot better than the day prior.

I was able to move out of the ICU room and was fortunate enough to move into a room by myself where I stayed for the remainder of my hospital stay. In my new room, I changed into my own clothes. It was a great feeling to get into my own pajamas and out of the hospital gown. I felt one step closer to heading home. A nurse named Malou cared for me while I was in this room. Just like the ICU nurses, she was warm and helpful and took great care of me. My son and my mom visited me at some point during the day, but I have no memory of their visit at all. I do remember Dr. Miller visiting to check on me and change my head dressing.

Aside from that, this second day was spent relaxing watching TV or listening to music, walking to and from the bathroom (holding the wall for support), and eating when my meals were delivered. I had brought a lot to the hospital that I never even touched, things like magazines and books. I was feeling good but wasn't bored or looking for any additional stimulation at all. I was experiencing very little pain and was hoping to be discharged the following day. I had an MRI that evening and can't remember much of it aside from how incredibly kind the men who assisted me through it were. Everyone I encountered at Mass Eye and Ear was wonderful.

I am very near-sighted and rely entirely on prescription glasses. I have difficulty wearing contact lenses, but I was required to wear that head dressing over my ear for five days post-surgery, which made wearing my glasses impossible. At the recommendation of my social media friends, I tried removing the right arm from an old pair of glasses, but that didn't work for me. They became so cock-eyed that my vision was even worse trying to wear glasses so crooked on my face. I ended up just not wearing glasses at all for that five-day period. That was an interesting experience, navigating the world through very blurry vision. Still, since it wasn't causing headaches, I just accepted it as the easiest solution to this temporary problem and lived sans glasses for a few days.

By the end of my second day in the hospital, I still hadn't had a visit from physical therapy. The doctors had ordered physical therapy since I was still quite unsteady on my feet. They wanted to make sure I was evaluated before I left the hospital to determine if vestibular therapy would be necessary. Since that didn't happen the second day, they were trying to coordinate it for the next morning and hoped I would be discharged and head home soon after.

That is exactly what happened. I saw a physical therapist the morning of my third day in the hospital. I had brought a cane with me to the hospital in case I needed it after surgery. She recommended that I use it for a while, and she took me for a walk around the hospital floor to observe how well I was able to move and use the cane. After our walk, she reminded me that unsteadiness is normal after this surgery, but I was doing great in these early days of recovery. She didn't think I would need vestibular therapy. Still, she gave me the name of a facility near my house in case I did need it in the future (depending on how I progressed and what Dr. Lee's recommendation was after seeing him for my two-week follow-up appointment). With the green light from the physical therapist, I was able to get clearance to be discharged and go home! I was nervous about going home where there would be no nurses, but I was also anxious to sleep in my own bed and be in my own space. This was especially true since I was lucky enough to have my period start that morning—it always shows up at the worst time—and I most wanted to be home in my own bed for the next several days.

Dr. Song visited me one last time and changed my head dressing again. Shortly after that, my mother and sister came to bring me home. By midday, I was in a wheelchair and leaving the hospital. And just like that, my surgery and hospitalization were over!

The surgery experience is such a difficult one to describe. Having no memory of the actual surgery is very bizarre. Knowing that my body endured such an invasive surgical procedure and having no memory of it, the time leading up to it, or the time immediately following it, is a strange feeling. It's like having no memory at all of the most important moment of your life, then waking up from it and just getting right to work on recovering and healing. Modern medicine is such a marvel to me after this experience.

Leaving the hospital was exciting and nerve-wracking. I had a very distinct feeling of a new beginning, a fresh start, an opportunity to live life without SCDS again (and appreciate it this time!)—but first, I had to get through the trip home. I had about a sixty-minute car ride ahead if we didn't hit traffic. This is much less travel than many SCDS patients must endure when getting home after surgery, but I was still anxious about it. The physical therapist had given me some tips for getting through travel, including keeping my eyes shut and being prepared to stop midway if I needed a break.

I was pleasantly surprised that my car ride home was quite easy. I didn't experience any motion sickness, and the dizziness wasn't any worse in the car than it was elsewhere at that point. I did have a travel neck pillow that I used for the car ride, and I was glad to have that. It helped me stay comfortable and keep my head relatively still. We were able to drive all the way home without having to stop for a break, other than the all-important pharmacy stop to pick up my plethora of prescriptions.

II WEEK 1: DID I EVEN HAVE SURGERY?

My first day or two home from the hospital was very strange. In hindsight, I believe it's because I now understand that anesthesia takes quite a while to fully work its way out of your body. I felt unbelievably good. If not for the glamorous head dressing, the dizziness and imbalance, and the miserable constipation (which I'll come back to), I wouldn't have even known I had surgery at all.

The hallmarks of my first week were boredom, pills, constipation, sleep, and my first peek at my incision. My second day home from the hospital, I was cutting potatoes in the kitchen, helping my mother make dinner, and asking her, "What the hell am I going to do for the next nine weeks?!" I was bored, if you can believe it. First of all, how sad is it that I really had been such a workaholic for so long that it only took four days (three of which were in a hospital) for me to be bored and wonder how I would ever fill my time without work? Secondly, how bizarre that I was feeling so well so early. This was nothing like what I was expecting my early days to be. I had been anticipating severe vertigo for weeks, plus severe pain from the craniotomy. I had neither.

My mother and sister mostly took care of me for the first two days. I had doctor's orders not to bend over, lift objects over five pounds, or drive. So basically, my options were to sit around all day and walk as much as possible. I still wasn't wearing my glasses, so television wasn't that engaging, and I had no desire at all to try to read a book yet. These early days were mostly spent talking with my mother, eating when hungry, and trying to walk once or twice a day. For the first few days, we walked just to the end of the driveway. After that, we'd venture a little farther with each walk, getting up to about a quarter of a mile in the first week. As far as eating, I could theoretically eat whatever I wanted, but I was experiencing tightness and soreness in my jaw. Prior to surgery, the kitchen had been stocked with soft foods so that I'd have options—soup, applesauce, ice cream, etc.

It took a while to adjust to all the medications I was taking —fourteen pills every morning! Some were required in the morning, others at night. Dr. Lee prescribed many for postoperative care, but some were my existing prescriptions. My mother and sister helped me figure out how many pills to take each day and when to take them. We ended up writing up a calendar schedule for each day and filling up plastic sandwich bags with pills. We had "am" bags and "pm" bags. Getting organized like this in the first couple of days ended up being a huge help, especially in the later days when I was home alone during my recovery. It was a total of nineteen days of post-operative medications, which included steroids, antivirals, Tylenol, stool softener, to name a few. I was prescribed a couple of days' worth of oxycodone for home, but I don't believe I ever took any oxycodone after I left the hospital. The extra strength Tylenol took care of the little pain I experienced. I did not want to mess up these medications and risk infection or adverse effects, so I recommend organizing the pills if you can.

I was on a high dosage of steroids that was keeping me awake, so I never napped at all during the day. I was expecting to be sleeping around the clock! Not the case at all. Sleep is precious to me. I definitely need my eight hours every night, or I'm grumpy. As a little girl, I was the one who would climb up onto my grandparents' couch and go to sleep when tired, instead of continuing to play with my cousins. I am a stomach sleeper, though, and I was instructed to sleep in an elevated position, which meant no stomach sleeping. Between that, the steroids, and the giant head dressing, I was nervous that sleep would be challenging. I requested permission to take Benadryl, so that was included in my evening pill regimen, and it did help. I was able to sleep through most or all the night every night, despite the early challenges.

Many friends online had recommended purchasing a wedge pillow or a reading pillow for sleeping elevated. I did get a reading pillow, but I also have an adjustable bed. I mostly used my adjustable bed to sleep in an elevated position, and that worked well for me after experimenting to find the right level of elevation. Once I found a reasonably comfortable position, I had no significant trouble falling or staying asleep.

I was able to get my first look at my incision and stitches during the first week. Even though my dressing had been changed twice during my hospital stay, I had never seen the surgical site. They never offered, and I never thought to ask. So, by the time the first five days had passed, I was excited to get my first look at my head and take my first shower.

My mother cut the bandages and removed the dressing from my head, and my first reaction was amazement at how heavy that dressing had been! I hadn't realized it until it was removed, but that was a weight on my head that I had been compensating for without realizing it. The second realization was how little hair had been shaved. If I hadn't told you they shaved part of my head, you'd never know it. My hair had to be pulled away from the incision to even be able to see it. The incision was easily identified by Dr. Lee's pristine handiwork. His approach to stitching must be rare because I've never seen surgery patients from another doctor look like Dr. Lee's stitches.

I had been told I could shower and wash my hair as soon as the dressing came off. I was nervous about this first shower but also really looking forward to it! Five days with no shower, plus my period? Hopefully, I'll never find myself in that situation again! I had a shower seat in my shower and was glad for it. I felt wobbly and weak in the shower and wasn't comfortable standing in there for more than a couple of minutes, but with the shower seat, I was able to take my time, being careful when working around my incision, and just relax in the shower. I washed very gingerly around the surgical site, still afraid to touch it. I mostly just ran the water over that side of my head and probably only washed half of my head.

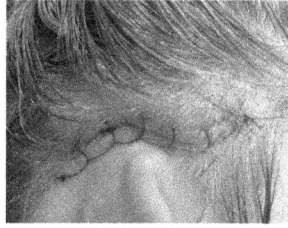

Once the dressing was off, I was able to start wearing my glasses. I could see again! That was a nice change. My incision was tucked so neatly behind my ear that my glasses didn't touch it much. I was able to wear my glasses directly over the incision without any gauze or anything.

In the first week, I relied on very simple supports to give myself comfort. I was surprised by how sore my throat was from being intubated during surgery, so I always kept cough drops nearby. They eased the throat discomfort. I also used ice packs to ease the pain in my jaw, especially after eating. After every meal, I would lie down under a weighted blanket for fifteen to thirty minutes and ice my jaw. Building intentional and regular self-care like this into my daily routines really helped me through these early days of recovery.

My biggest troubles in this first week were in the bathroom! Despite starting stool softeners in the hospital and continuing a healthy daily dose of them at home, I reached the end of my first week and still had no bowel movement and grew more uncomfortable with each passing day. I laugh at that now because it's so incredible to me that doctors could screw a hole in my skull, and the worst part of it all was not being able to go to the bathroom afterward! It was all very surreal. My grandmother was calling every day to check on me, and it quickly became a joke that her first question was always whether I had finally been able to poop! And when the first week ended, I still hadn't gone and was becoming pretty miserable about it.

III WEEK 2: EUREKA!

On day nine, when I was so uncomfortable with constipation that I was losing any desire to eat and I was contemplating whether I should call Dr. Lee's office, my mother told me to go for a walk around the house. So, I started doing laps around the kitchen and living room. Ten minutes later, I walked back into my bedroom exclaiming, "I did it"!

"Did what?" my mom replied.

"I pooped!"

"Ha! That was fast," she laughed.

Eureka! The phrase *relieve yourself* suddenly made a lot more sense to me. I was definitely relieved! I wasn't allowed to physically exert myself yet, but I felt like jumping for joy. Week two was off to a great start.

But constipation is no joke. I honestly don't know what I could have done differently to avoid this problem (and the diarrhea I then dealt with for the next day or two), but I strongly suggest everyone have a conversation with their surgeon *before* surgery to understand how to best prepare to get your bowels moving again quickly after surgery!

The second week was full of *Eureka!* moments like this. At some point during the second week, I was able to walk a half-mile for the first time. I was still using a cane outside of the house, but when walking around inside, I was able to get around no problem without my cane. I had visits from my best friends and visited a couple of stores as well. It was a remarkable experience, and no one—me especially—could believe how well I was doing. I thought I'd be bed-bound for weeks after having a craniotomy, suffering from pain and vertigo. My actual experience was nothing like that, though. It was all so surreal.

The biggest *Eureka!* moment of them all, though, was during week two. I was home alone, and it was raining. I decided to try reading for the first time since surgery to see what that felt like. After a few minutes of reading, it suddenly dawned on me that all I could hear was the rain. I could not hear my eyeballs moving! I could not hear my heart beating! Oh, the triumph I experienced can't even be described. All I could do was cry—happy, joyful, wonderful tears of freedom and hope. The rain was tranquil. My bed was warm and comforting. My freshly shaved legs were smooth against my sheets. All my senses were alive in a totally new way. The future felt limitless. I cried for a long time that night. My body and mind felt so connected, and so at peace, more so than ever in my life before now. This exact moment is what I had been waiting for, and working toward, for two years. And here it was. I was in it.

IV WEEKS 3 & 4: RECOVERY REALITIES

It wasn't until the third week that I actually started feeling like I had had surgery. I was still sleeping in an elevated position, my body felt weak, my stitches were itchy, I was dizzy all the time, my head felt numb and uncomfortable around the incision, and all the medication I was choking down morning and evening was getting old. I was swallowing fourteen pills every morning and almost as many at night. It would take me up to an hour to sit in bed and force them all down (yes, I'm a wimp about swallowing pills). A lot of those pills were the 60 mg of Prednisone I was taking. Steroids are known to have unpleasant side effects. For me, that was true. I had difficulty sleeping, so I was taking a sleep-aid every night to make sure I rested overnight. During the day, I never napped while taking steroids. Not even once. That's unbelievable for someone like me, who can practically sleep on-demand, anywhere, any time, and who had required a nap every day for most of the last two years! Suddenly, I was awake more than asleep, and this was a huge change in my life post-surgery. Some of the Prednisone side effects were harder, though. My heart was *pounding* all the time, and I was jittery and shaky like I was hopped up on caffeine.

None of this was pleasant, but I reminded myself every day that these were temporary challenges. I knew I would be able to stop taking the steroids someday soon and that getting through the surgery recovery was not supposed to be easy or quick. Reminding myself it was temporary became an important daily thought. A few weeks of steroid side effects was a sacrifice I was more than willing to make.

In my third week of recovery, I had an appointment to see Dr. Lee for a checkup and to have my stitches removed. I could not wait to see Dr. Lee! I felt like he and his team had given me back an opportunity to live. It's a feeling so immense I can barely begin to describe it. This one doctor and his team made the difference between a lifetime of imprisonment to this horrible condition and a life of freedom, opportunity, and restored health. I was excited to see him and tell him. But the drive into Boston was not something I was looking forward to. I had only spent a few minutes in the car at a time and was always very dizzy, so I didn't know what to expect while driving in and out of Boston, a city famous for its traffic.

The drive sucked. By the time we finally got to Mass Eye and Ear, I was very dizzy and having motion sickness, nausea, and headache. My mother had driven me to the appointment since I wasn't able to drive yet. While we waited for Dr. Lee, she tried to make casual conversation. My responses were short, and I stayed mostly silent. Eventually, she turned and asked me, "Are you okay? You seem more nervous now than you did before the surgery." I wasn't nervous at all, but I was feeling so dizzy and sick that I couldn't do much but sit there and wait. This put a damper on my time with Dr. Lee because I just didn't feel well enough to engage with him and ask questions like I had hoped. Nonetheless, the appointment had some exciting highlights!

Dr. Lee did the tuning fork test during this appointment. If you remember from earlier, when I was sick with SCDS, the tuning fork screamed in my right ear like a fire alarm and made the room go sideways. So, when I saw him pull out his tuning fork, I shrank at the site of it—but then he held it to my forehead, and nothing happened. Nothing happened! No fire alarm. No vertigo. I was overcome with emotion and found myself choking back tears. *How could it be? Just three weeks ago, this test would've knocked me on my ass, but here I was, post-surgery with no reaction at all. Maybe I really was cured!* Something about Dr. Lee's reaction to this made me wonder if he was nervous that I had some hearing loss since I wasn't hearing anything at all on the right side when he used the tuning fork. I pushed that thought immediately out of my mind, though, because this was a monumental moment, and I felt like I was hearing just fine in my right ear. *Wow. Life post-SCDS really was a possibility. And I had already started living it. What a gift.*

Dr. Lee assured me my daily dizziness was totally normal at this point. He reminded me several times that I *just* had major surgery. He was glad to hear I was already walking a half-mile each day and said I could drive when I felt ready. I didn't feel ready yet but was glad to know I could try as soon as I felt up to it. This was also the day that I would begin my steroid taper, meaning I'd finally be done taking the steroids soon. Dr. Lee wrapped up the appointment by explaining I'd see him again when I hit the three-month mark. This would be to repeat my hearing and VEMP testing, then meet with him to review the test results together.

That night I was home alone. My boyfriend and I had split up, and my son was now in college. My mother was my primary caretaker after surgery, but she slept most nights at her own house because I was feeling well enough to sleep overnight on my own, and she deserved to be in her own bed. Anyway, as I lay in bed that night, I suddenly heard the faint *boom boom boom* of my heartbeat in my ear. I froze in disbelief. There was no way that I had seen Dr. Lee this morning and told him all my auditory symptoms were gone, only to have pulsatile tinnitus return that very night. In my mind, I went right back to those early days—denying the noise in my ear, pushing it to the background, telling myself it wasn't real.

The next day, I woke up and could still hear it: *boom boom boom* in my right ear. It was quiet, but it was there. The effect on my mood was palpable. My anxiety peaked immediately. I was so worried that this was the beginning of a terrible journey back into SCDS. This whole experience was such a roller coaster, with almost constant ups and downs. It has been like whiplash.

So, I took the question to my SCDS friends on social media. I had been posting weekly updates to the group to share my surgery experience because I wanted to give back to the group as much as I had received from it. That group never lets me down, and this was no exception. When I mentioned that my pulsatile tinnitus had returned, a friend commented to say that it could be a result of beginning my taper off the steroids. Apparently, it's common for some swelling to return when we stop the steroids, and that swelling could lead to the temporary return of some symptoms. I clung to this idea like a life preserver and reminded myself to be patient with my recovery in the hopes that my pulsatile tinnitus would eventually go away again. After all, it had only been three weeks since they drilled a hole in my skull. I knew I needed to give myself time and remain as relaxed as possible.

I set out to establish a daily routine that would support my recovery and overall wellbeing at the same time. This was the first significant break from work I had ever taken in my life. Even after giving birth, I was home with my son for less than two months before returning to college full-time.

I didn't want to waste this opportunity to experience deep rest for the first time ever. It didn't take long to realize, though, that I wasn't going to be capable of lying around watching TV all day, and I had made an iron-clad promise to myself to stay out of my work email no matter what. This was *my* time, and I wanted to completely disconnect from work and figure out who I was—without work and without SCDS. I wasn't thinking of my surgery recovery as just physical healing. This was my chance to process all the transitions life was throwing at me and listen to my intuition to forge my path forward.

My son was now a high school graduate, so our relationship was changing quickly, and I was struggling with it. For the first time in my adult life, I was grappling with the idea of putting myself first and supporting my son's independence. I was still grieving the loss of my dog six months prior, who passed away just two weeks after my son moved out to start college. It was like losing all my kids at the same time. Also, my partner and I were preparing to sell our home, which meant moving into a new place by myself just weeks after my surgery. I had some big questions about work to consider, as well—how to make the most of my current position and how to get myself back to working as a therapist as well. This recovery was more like a rebirth. I could choose to see my future as uncertain and scary or limitless and entirely up to me. My next chapter could be determined by me, for me, my own wants and needs. What family, friends, or society thought I should do wouldn't be my top concern anymore. I was going to listen only to myself because SCDS had taught me that I knew what was best.

Despite my high hopes for these ten weeks at home, I was bored quickly. TV and movies didn't hold my attention; documentaries were super depressing, and, with the sustained dizziness, I wasn't motivated to read any of my books or magazines. So, I went back to the wellness wheel to see how I might be able to utilize it while I was recovering. What resonated with me most was a desire to pursue my spiritual and intellectual needs.

Most mornings, I was nauseous for a bit after taking all my medications, so I watched a documentary about Buddhism every morning after breakfast. Then I would take a walk and then meditate. By the time I finished my morning routine, it was usually time for lunch. Using my mornings to learn, move my body, and quiet my mind became a daily ritual that allowed me to remain patient and calm through the natural ups and downs of recovery and get used to amplifying my intuitive voice to guide me forward.

V WEEKS 5-10: WAKING UP AGAIN

Before I knew it, an entire month had passed since my surgery. For the most part, my recovery felt remarkable. I mean, it really felt like a miracle. It was so hard to believe it was real. However, I did still have some not-so-good days. My not-so-good days sometimes had a physical cause; other times they were more psychological. One of the frustrations of living with SCDS is the ups and downs, where you'll have a string of good days and almost convince yourself you aren't sick anymore, followed by a string of bad days where you are all but bedridden. I found recovering from surgery to be similar but with less variance between the good and bad. Overall, I was exponentially better than I had been before surgery. The not-so-good days were still there, though.

SCDS experts in the medical field are very clear that surgery patients should expect dizziness after surgery. I knew it was coming, but I wasn't entirely sure what to expect, which made me fearful. It's one of the reasons so many SCDS sufferers, especially those like me who suffer from primarily auditory symptoms, are hesitant to commit to surgery. My experience with dizziness after surgery has most certainly been worse than any dizziness I encountered before surgery. And yet, I'd choose surgery again and again.

The cumulative effect of *all* the symptoms I was trying to live with before surgery was far and away more miserable and more debilitating than the dizziness I've faced since surgery. This is true for the pulsatile tinnitus that returned after surgery as well. Before my MFC, I was always hearing my heartbeat; it ranged in volume from a whisper to a scream. When it returned three weeks after surgery, I could only hear it sometimes, only two or three days per week, and it was always a whisper.

The impact of these physical symptoms was connected to the psychological changes that I noticed after surgery. I feared that my surgery had failed and SCDS was coming back. After all, dizziness and pulsatile tinnitus *are* SCDS symptoms. I felt good but noticed I was holding myself back from fully acknowledging it. I was afraid it wouldn't last, that I would wake up one day and find myself pulled back into the SCDS nightmare with all the noise and all the pain, exhaustion, and solitude. But everyone kept telling me it was too early to know the surgery results.

I heard Dr. Lee in my head, reminding me that I *just* had major surgery, and suddenly it dawned on me that I wasn't struggling with SCDS anymore. What I was doing now was recovering from surgery! It was a confusing experience because the dizziness and pulsatile tinnitus were some of my SCDS symptoms before surgery, but when I stopped to think deeply about it, I realized that I was not experiencing these symptoms now as a sign of SCDS. Instead, they were a sign that my body was healing from surgery. My newly plugged ear canal meant that my system was learning how to function with two canals working in my right ear instead of three, and my surgery site was still healing, and likely swollen, which could easily explain the occasional pulsatile tinnitus.

Instead of focusing on the fear that my SCDS could return, I focused on this new reality I was experiencing. I felt a million times better than I had before surgery. That was real. I deserved to believe that I was on my way to being healthy again (just like I deserved to hunt down a diagnosis when I knew something was wrong with me) and allow myself to start healing psychologically from the trauma of living with SCDS. After working so hard to believe that I was truly sick, now my job was to work equally hard to believe that I was healthy again. This is how I channeled my energy for the next couple of months until I saw Dr. Lee again and had my post-operative testing done.

I remained committed to my daily morning ritual: a documentary about Buddhism, a walk, and a meditation. By now, I was able to walk an entire mile, and when the weather was nice, I would do that twice per day. I could tell the walking had increased my balance and decreased my dizziness by a lot. In the fifth week, I had ditched my cane, no longer needing any additional support while walking. Soon after, I began driving short distances.

Around this time, I noticed myself disconnecting from my SCDS groups on social media. I had a strong desire to stop thinking about SCDS altogether, to purge myself of that identity, and live a life completely void of SCDS. I felt bad about this because I knew that my success story was important to my peers on social media, but it didn't even feel like a choice to stop interacting online. It was a need. I began focusing on the things I was excited about adding to my new life post-SCDS.

I noticed a new feeling blossoming deep inside of me, like I was waking up for the first time in a long time. My body and mind, which had been using all available energy just to drag myself around every day, were suddenly more awake and alive. A desire to really live again was making its way to the surface. In response to this new energy I felt, I developed a new afternoon routine to add to my morning ritual. My brain was beginning to feel ready for work again, but I was not going to open my work email and get sucked into that world before it was time. Instead, I began pursuing two long-term goals I had set a while ago but could never quite find the time or energy for.

There was a counseling training I wanted to complete so that I could earn a specific credential. I purchased the course materials and spent some time each day beginning these studies. I had also always dreamed about writing a book (and you're reading the result of that dream right now!). I knew the world of SCDS patients and their loved ones needed more resources, and I thought I could help. Before my surgery, I had written an article that was very well received by my SCDS friends, so I knew I could use that article as the starting point for my book. I also started dedicating a portion of each day to writing or brainstorming what I thought would need to be included in the book and what message I hoped to deliver. This was my first time ever pursuing "work" purely because I wanted to, without any consideration for how these new pursuits might impact me financially, professionally, or as a mother. I was working on these projects purely because I was interested in them.

Those remaining weeks of my recovery were some of the most physically and mentally healing and productive of my life. I followed my daily routine for many weeks and even moved out of my house right in the middle of all this. And through it all, I continued to hit notable milestones in my recovery.

I celebrated Mother's Day with my family, tried my first alcoholic beverage since surgery, and encountered no negative side effects from the alcohol. No autophony. No vertigo. I began adapting to loud noise again, as well. I knew it would take some time for me to see our noisy world as a safe place again, but the difference was clear already. I was much less jumpy around unexpected noise and had no trouble in loud places like restaurants. I was still carrying earplugs with me but hadn't even used them once since my surgery. I even completed a two-hour hike through the woods ten weeks after my surgery! It was clear to me that I was not suffering with SCDS anymore and that I could move on with my life now.

I returned to work full-time ten weeks after my craniotomy and stepped into my life after SCDS. It was the same life I had put on pause to pursue surgery (in the hopes of healing), but now everything was different. I wasn't the same person I had been ten weeks ago.

The timing of when SCDS took over my life, forcing me inward to understand myself and my needs better, is fascinating to me now in retrospect. I was entering a time in my life when I was transitioning into independent adulthood for the first time. With my son growing up, my dog passing away, and my relationship ending, I found myself thrust into a world where it wasn't just normal, but it was necessary to put myself first. I was untethered from so many of the responsibilities that had ruled my existence for so long.

I often wonder how different my journey would have been if I had become sick with SCDS when my son was younger. I'm fearful I would have ignored my declining health for a very long time and lived a miserable life. It is undeniable that somehow the universe delivers to us the lessons we need at the exact moment in time we are ready to learn from them.

My life without SCDS is still in the early days, and so is my intuitive life. Do I wish I could have learned these lessons without having two years of suffering and a craniotomy? Hell, yes! I wish I was "untamed,"[1] as Glennon Doyle says, at a much earlier age. I mostly wish I had raised my son to listen to his intuition and know that he is innately wise, instead of modeling for him a need to strive for societal ideals that may or may not align with his heart. He's a young man now, but I know he's still watching me from a distance. Now I hope he'll notice that I've abandoned my scarlet letter. I've abandoned the need for redemption because I didn't do anything wrong. I did something great when I made my family. As I step into tomorrow, the only goal I carry is noticing what makes my heart race, endlessly pursuing authenticity even when it feels scary, and, well, turning into me. Only me. It's my own life to live.

VI BEGIN AGAIN

About a month after returning to work, it was time to see Dr. Lee again! This time for my three-month checkup, which would include a hearing test, a VEMP test, and a meeting with Dr. Lee. When he entered the room, he gave me his customary fist-bump greeting and asked me how I was. "Great! I think I'm cured," I replied as he turned to his monitor and started reading my test results. "I think you are too," he said.

He then walked me through the hearing and VEMP test results, explaining that all my results showed evidence that the surgery was successful. Where I used to be able to hear sound below zero decibels, this recent hearing test (below) showed that I wasn't hearing below zero anymore, and there was no indication of hearing loss.

FREQUENCY (Hz)

	125	250	500	1000	2000	4000	8000	16k

HEARING LEVEL (dB) ANSI 1969

dB	R	L
SDT:		
SRT:	7	7
PTA:	10	10

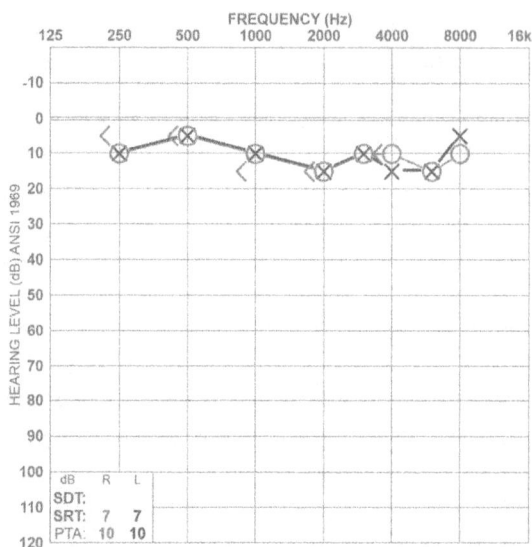

The VEMP test also showed improved results, what he would expect to see after an MFC. Having this physical evidence that I didn't have SCDS anymore was just as monumental a moment as when I first saw evidence that I *did* have SCDS. I asked Dr. Lee about my continued dizziness and the numbness I was still feeling on the right side of my head. Calm as ever, he explained that one or both could be permanent, or they could slowly resolve themselves over time. All I could do was wait and see. And that was just fine by me! Are there moments when I wish I could have no dizziness? Of course, but this is my reality right now, and it's okay. I have some minor dizziness each day, but it does not interfere with my functioning or overall wellbeing. I'm healthy. I do not have SCDS. I don't need much more.

As Dr. Lee wrapped up our conversation, he said we would schedule another round of testing in one year. There was a mini explosion in my head when he said he didn't expect me to require any further care for an entire year! Incredible.

I stepped out of the hospital into the warm summer air, knowing I wouldn't be back here for a long time. I tilted my head back, squinting into the sunlight, and really looked at the hospital for the first time. This was the place I lived for a few days. The place where Dr. Lee and his team gifted me the miracle of their brilliant talent. The city noise and the ambulance sirens caused me no pain. The crumbling side-walks were not a challenge for my now-steady gait. The drive home would not make me ill. I walked into that hospital with SCDS, and I was walked out without it. I don't want to face a journey like SCDS again, but should I have to, something tells me I can.

EPILOGUE

Here I am, one year after surgery. I remain thankful beyond words to Dr. Lee for giving me my life back. I'm also awakening to the reality that, in a variety of ways, some psychological and some physical, I will always carry traces of SCDS with me. I have some minor dizziness and quiet pulsatile tinnitus sometimes. Neither disrupts my daily life. Both remind me that I've survived every challenge I've faced so far and that, using my intuition and skills for wellness to guide me forward, I'll continue on. One day at a time.

NOTES

1. SICK

1. A classic American novel by Nathaniel Hawthorne, *The Scarlet Letter* tells the story of Hester who suffers public shame and shunning (in the form of a scarlet letter "A" she is forced to wear on her breast) as punishment for the supposedly "sinful" circumstances surrounding the birth of her child.
2. https://www.ata.org/about-tinnitus/
3. *Miller-Keane Encyclopedia and Dictionary of Medicine, Nursing, and Allied Health, Seventh Edition.* S.v. "autophony." Retrieved February 4 2023 from https://medical-dictionary.thefreedictionary.com/autophony
4. BBC News. 2011. "Man Cured of Hearing His Eyeballs Move," July 27, 2011, sec. Oxford. https://www.bbc.com/news/uk-england-oxford-shire-14308474.

3. SURVIVAL

1. https://nationalwellness.org/resources/six-dimensions-of-wellness/
2. https://mfpcc.samhsa.gov/ENewsArticles/Article12b_2017.aspx

4. TREATMENT

1. https://doctors.masseyeandear.org/details/125

5. HEALING

1. Doyle, Glennon. 2020. Untamed. National Geographic Books.

APPENDIX A – SUICIDE RESOURCES

National Suicide Lifeline (United States)

- Call or text 988
- https://988lifeline.org

International Suicide Resources

- International Association for Suicide Prevention (https://www.iasp.info)
- Suicide Awareness Voices of Education (SAVE) (https:save.org/find-help/international-resources)

APPENDIX B – A LIST OF SCDS SYMPTOMS WITH A SENSE OF HUMOR

Roger Campbell, a wise and kind SCDS warrior with an incredible sense of humor, created the following list of SCDS symptoms for those looking to gain better understanding of the condition. When he shares this list on social media, Roger is always careful to point out that you don't need to experience all these symptoms to have SCDS and, of course, proper diagnosis requires the care of a medical doctor.

1. Do you have tinnitus?

2. Do you have a feeling of fullness in one ear, like someone has shoved a wine cork in there?

3. Do you experience virtually constant dizziness, aggravated by straining or exertion?

4. Is your own voice amplified and distorted inside your head, generally on one side?

5. When emptying the dishwasher, does the sound of two dinner plates hitting each other feel like an ice pick being shoved through your eardrum into your brain?

6. Do sudden sharp low-pitched sounds make the room "move"?

7. Does eating a mouthful of corn chips sound like your house is being demolished with you in it?

8. Does humming the national anthem sound unbearably distorted?

9. Do you have trouble walking on uneven surfaces—particularly in low light?

10. In a quiet room, can you hear yourself blink and can you hear your eyeballs move?

11. Borrow a tuning fork, strike it, and place it in the middle of your forehead. Is it louder in one ear? In more advanced cases, you will be able to hear it in your bad ear when placed on your sternum, shoulder bone, hip, and even ankle bone. You can also turn on the kitchen faucet and put your forehead on the kitchen counter, and again, is the noise louder in one ear?

12. When you run, does the whole world bounce?

13. Do you have trouble hearing people talk in a moderately noisy environment?

14. There's a protrusion of cartilage in front of your ear hole. Gently push it back so it seals the ear canal airtight. Gently at first, pump the sealed ear canal. Does the room jump with each push?

15. Can you hear your heartbeat?

16. Do you have trouble watching a video clip on a smart-phone while standing up?

17. Do you have memory problems?

18. Do you suffer from neck and shoulder stiffness?

19. Do you walk a bit like a duck?

20. Do you sleep (or want to sleep) abnormally long hours?

21. Do you get earaches (usually on one side)?

22. Do you get the form of vertigo that feels like there's a sack of flour pushing down on the top of your head?

APPENDIX C – SOME STRATEGIES FOR LIVING WITH SCDS

- Connect with peers. There are two groups on Facebook for SCDS patients and their loved ones: "SCDS Support (Superior Canal Dehiscence Syndrome)" and "Superior Canal Dehiscence Syndrome Support Group (SCDS)"
- Teach the people close to you the name of SCDS, what it means, and what your life is like with SCDS
- Seek medical care from an SCDS expert, and advocate for your needs
- Listen to your body, and let it guide you forward
- Use phone apps like the Calm app for meditation and mindfulness
- Try to engage in daily activity like a short walk (as much as reasonable, without pushing yourself too hard)
- Control the noise in your home environment: turn off the TV surround sound, listen to quiet music as a distraction, replace heavy dinnerware with

plastic/lightweight alternatives, use closed captions on the TV with low volume

- Don't overextend yourself, and when you have a busy day, plan a day for rest the next day
- Identify your limitations, and set boundaries with your loved ones
- Say no to things you know you can't do
- Seek medical accommodations with your employer
- Give yourself permission to move slower than you might have before
- Ask for help!
- Find earplugs that are comfortable for you, and use those when you can't avoid a noisy environment
- When flying, use "earplanes" earplugs (found on Amazon or at your local retailer)
- Monitor barometric pressure, and prepare for low-pressure days; free apps such as WeatherX and Barometer Plus are available
- Study Buddhism and/or mindfulness
- Set realistic expectations for what you'll accomplish each day
- Treat each day like a new day
- If you are experiencing symptoms of depression and/or anxiety, seek counseling with a licensed therapist, and consider discussing medication options with your physician

APPENDIX D – RESOURCES THAT HELPED ME LEARN, SURVIVE, AND THRIVE

MEDICAL WEBSITES:

Cleveland Clinic

- https://my.clevelandclinic.org/health/diseases/15266-superior-canal-dehiscence-scd

Johns Hopkins Medicine

- https://www.hopkinsmedicine.org/health/conditions-and-diseases/superior-canal-dehiscence-syndrome-scds
- https://www.hopkinsmedicine.org/otolaryngology/specialty_areas/otology/conditions/superior-canal-dehiscence-syndrome/

Mass General Brigham & Mass Eye and Ear

- https://www.masseyeandear.org/conditions/superior-semicircular-canal-dehiscence-syndrome
- https://www.brighamandwomensfaulkner.org/programs-and-services/otolaryngology/ear/superior-semicircular-canal-dehiscence

UCLA

- https://www.uclahealth.org/neurosurgery/semicircular-canal-dehiscence

OTHER WEBSITES:

National Organization for Rare Disorders

- https://rarediseases.org/rare-diseases/superior-semicircular-canal-dehiscence/

The Mighty

- https://themighty.com

Vestibular Disorders Association (VeDA)

- https://vestibular.org

BOOKS:

- *A Hole in My Life. Battling Chronic Dizziness* by Philippa Thomson

- *No Nonsense Buddhism for Beginners* by Noah Rasheta
- *The Book of Joy: Lasting Happiness in a Changing World* by His Holiness the Dalai Lama, Archbishop Desmond Tutu, with Douglas Abrams
- *Untamed* by Glennon Doyle
- *You Are Here* by Thich Nhat Hahn

PODCASTS

- *Secular Buddhism* hosted by Noah Rasheta
- *Buddhism Boot Camp* hosted by Timber Hawkeye
- *Dare to Lead* hosted by Brene Brown
- *Intuitive Girls Guide* hosted by Jamie Hayhurst and Heather Wood
- *Ten Percent Happier* hosted by Dan Harris
- *We Can Do Hard Things* hosted by Glennon Doyle

APPENDIX E – SCDS QUESTIONS TO ASK YOUR DOCTOR

This list of questions was compiled from the amazing SCDS communities on social media where "What should I ask the doctor?" is one of the most common posts. This is an exhaustive list of questions. Some will apply to you; others may not. You likely won't ask your doctor every question, or all at once, but you'll have a sense of what to be aware of through your journey.

BEFORE SURGERY

- Which surgery/surgeries do you perform? How do you determine which procedure to use for each individual patient?
- How often have you performed the surgery? What is the success rate?
- What are the risks associated with surgery?
- What are the odds of full recovery?

- What are the odds some of my symptoms won't be cured by surgery? Which symptoms?
- What are the odds of an infection after surgery?
- How many people require revision surgery?
- What's an average recovery time (returning to work, driving, caring for kids, etc.)?
- Get a detailed explanation of the procedure – Transmastoid (TM) or Middle Fossa Craniotomy (MFC), plugging and/or resurfacing? What are the pros and cons of each and why?
- Can you estimate how large my dehiscence is?
- Where is my dehiscence located, and does that make the surgery more complicated?
- How will the surgery impact my vestibular system? Should I expect dizziness after surgery and, if so, temporarily or permanently?
- Do I need a COVID test before surgery? If so, how many days ahead?
- What process do I follow with your office staff to get all employer paperwork completed ahead of my medical leave?
- If seeking surgery out of state, ask about travel guidelines & expectations before surgery
- If bilateral, how many people require surgery on both sides? How soon after can the second surgery be scheduled? Should I expect my other ear to get worse after I have the first surgery?

DURING SURGERY

- How long should I expect the surgery to last?

- What exactly does the surgery entail? Where is the incision & how large?
- How will the surgeon navigate to the inner ear (cut through jaw muscle, etc.)?
- How much of my head will be shaved?
- What material is used for closing the dehiscence?
- How is the surgical site closed (titanium plate, mesh, screws, staples, stitches, etc.)?
- What to expect from the time I arrive at the hospital through the time I'm discharged?
- How long will I be in the hospital? Will I be in the ICU?

AFTER SURGERY

- What's the average recovery look like?
- What's the infection rate?
- Any difficulties to expect after surgery?
- What kind of pain management should I expect after surgery (what kind of prescription meds, for how long, etc.)? Should I anticipate side effects?
- How long until I can do everyday things, such as: wash my hair, bending/lifting, sex, drive, return to work?
- How soon after surgery should I expect to see you?
- How many times will I see you when I'm in the hospital?
- How should I expect to feel when I wake up from surgery?
- What are the odds of nausea/vomiting after surgery? Could that impact the surgery results?

- Will surgery cause any of my symptoms to seem worse/unresolved when I wake up from anesthesia (due to inflammation, fluid, etc.)?
- Knowing SCDS surgeries sometimes fail, what should I be watching out for?
- What follow-up care should I expect after leaving the hospital? When will I see you again, and will we have regular appointments? If so, on what schedule?
- What signs do I look out for that might signal something is wrong after surgery?
- What do I do if I am concerned that something doesn't feel right and I think I need an emergency assessment after surgery?
- What testing should I expect after surgery and when (hearing, VEMP, etc.)?
- If seeking surgery out of state, ask about travel guidelines & expectations after surgery
- What rehabilitation planning is recommended? Will I get a list of exercises to do daily and/or be referred for physical or vestibular therapy?

APPENDIX F – HELPFUL STRATEGIES & SUPPLIES FOR SURGERY AND RECOVERY

Again, this list was compiled by reviewing the many posts in SCDS social media groups where helpful items are often shared by SCDS patients.

For Hospital

- Grip socks so I don't have to wear what the hospital gives me
- Blanket from home
- Travel neck pillow
- Black-out eye mask
- Comfortable earplugs/earbuds for music
- Child's toothbrush
- Pajamas (bring an extra set just in case)
- Cane

For Home

- Jaw ice pack (a cold wrap for jaw/wisdom teeth pain)
- Wedge pillow or reading pillow
- Travel neck pillow
- Cane
- Cough drops
- Weighted blanket
- A daily calendar of required pills, for am and pm
- A daily routine for keeping your mind and body active
- Morning and afternoon walk (starting very short, gradually adding distance)
- Morning or afternoon stimulation: reading, meditation, watching a documentary, hosting a visitor, coloring, knitting, or anything that you find fun and stimulating

APPENDIX G – NATIONAL TEMPORAL BONE REGISTRY

https://masseyeandear.org/tbregistry

What SCDS patients need the most is an increased understanding of the condition. One way to help us get there is to join the National Temporal Bone Registry.

In 1992, the National Institute on Deafness and Other Communication Disorders (NIDCD) established the National Temporal Bone Registry. It is housed at Mass Eye and Ear in Boston, MA. The registry's goal is to research the auditory and vestibular systems and learn more about causes and cures for conditions like SCDS. Visit the link above to learn more and find instructions to join the registry.

APPENDIX H – SOME PHOTOS OF MY SURGERY JOURNEY

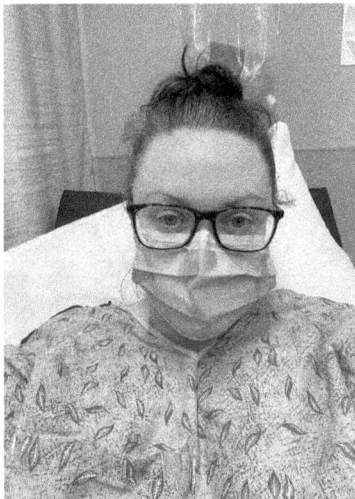

Pre-operative care on surgery day

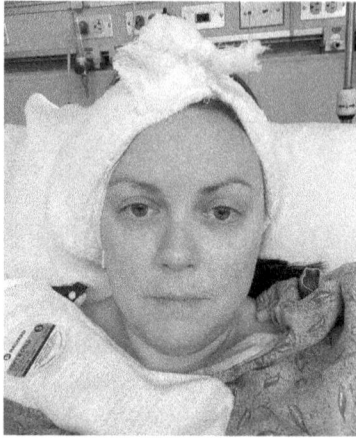

Day after surgery

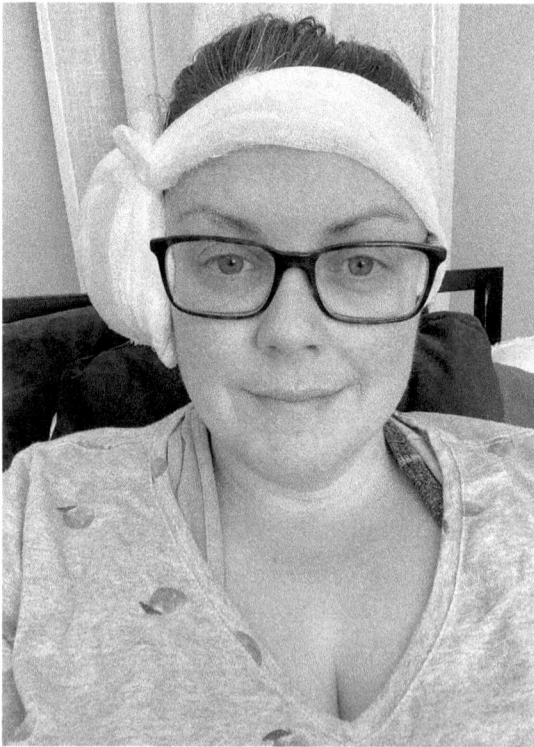

Five days after surgery, about to take the head dressing off!

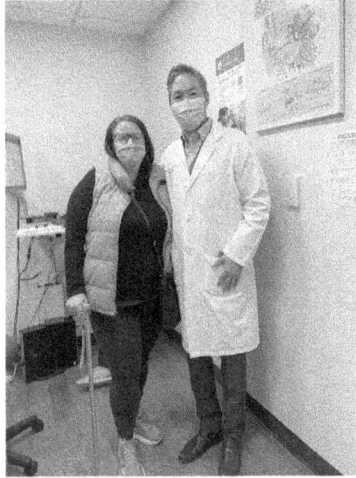

Three weeks post-op visit with Dr. Lee!

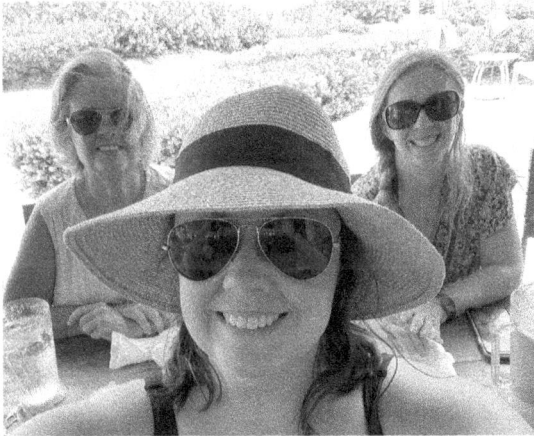

Six months post-op, enjoying a girls' weekend in Puerto Rico with my mother and sister and living a normal life again!

ACKNOWLEDGMENTS

I would like to acknowledge all the SCDS warriors out there, especially the many friends and cheerleaders I've met in our Facebook groups. Special thanks to Carissa Pichon and Roger Campbell for their contributions to this book.

I am a strong woman, thanks to the equally strong women I get to share this life with. To the best friends a girl could ask for, Sandy Rodricks and Heather Wood, thank you for helping me trust my intuition and for being by my side through all of life's ups and downs. To my Nanny, Ann Packard, thank you for giving me my love of books, for serving up lots of "TLC" when I was unwell, and for being the first to read this manuscript. I'd like to thank my sisters, Katie Langton, Erin Folloni, and Tiffany Kowarsky, and my aunts, Marybeth Hammond and Sarah Packard, for supporting me through my recovery. And to my mom, Lisa Drew, the woman who drove to my house just to hug me on the day I was finally diagnosed and whose enduring support could never be described in words. Thank you for teaching me to live a life dedicated to helping others.

I would also like to thank Noah Rasheta for supporting me, and so many others, on the path to enlightenment through his ministry and wisdom.

To Sigrid Macdonald and Andrea Schmidt, who gave their editing and design expertise to this project, thank you for making my vision a reality.

To those I have loved and lost much too soon—Amy, Skylur, Grandpa Ralph, Grandpa Mike, Chris, and Booker —your memory and spirit comforted me through the fear I faced on this journey.

Last, thank you to Dr. Daniel Lee and the entire staff at Boston's Mass Eye and Ear Infirmary for giving me my life back.

ABOUT THE AUTHOR

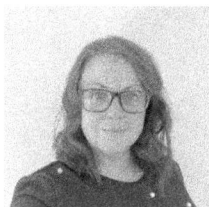

Lauren Folloni is a university administrator and social worker. In her free time, she enjoys reading, volunteering, studying Buddhism, and daydreaming about traveling the world someday. She loves spending time with family and friends, especially her nieces and nephews. She's dedicated to raising awareness of invisible illness, especially SCDS. She lives with her son in southeastern Massachusetts.

Reach out: www.laurenfolloni.com
@laurenfolloni

www.ingramcontent.com/pod-product-compliance
Lightning Source LLC
LaVergne TN
LVHW041321080426
835513LV00008B/535